Questioning Protocol

by
Randi Redmond Oster

First Edition. Printed in the United States of America.

Book design by Vox One: www.voxone.com

Distributed by Atlas Books
www.atlasbooks.com
800.247.6553 or 800.266.5564

ISBN 978-0-9899120-0-6
ISBN Paperback: 978-0-9899120-0-6
978-0-9899120-1-3 (ePUB)
978-0-9899120-2-0 (ePDF)
Library of Congress Control Number: 2013949300

For more information:
Well Path Press
2860 North Street
Fairfield, CT 06824
www.wellpathpress.com

10 9 8 7 6 5 4 3 2 1

Disclosure: To protect their privacy, I have changed the names of most people in this book, including all doctors. I have not altered the names of family members, Gary Kempinski and Mark Grashow, among a few others.

Disclaimer: The information in this book is not intended or implied to be a substitute for professional medical advice, diagnosis or treatment. All content, including text, graphics, images and information, contained in or available through this book is for general information purposes only.

*To my wonderful husband, Steve,
whose love, support and belief in me
have made my dreams come true.*

Table of Contents

Chapter 1

From Fumes to Flowers

"Let's go to Wild Rice for lunch, Mom," Gary, my 15-year-old, too-skinny son insists before he even sits down in the car and closes the door. I start driving before my son belts in; otherwise the other moms will start honking. I am in the high school pick-up lane and Gary just finished taking the PSAT, a test that predicts college placement. I bet it is high anxiety day for all these high school parents, waiting in line like me. We're in Fairfield, on the gold coast of Connecticut, a place where status and college and money seem to be key measurements of success. I'm afraid I've become a reluctant participant.

We live a lovely lifestyle in a 4,000-square-foot colonial on two acres with a heated pool and garden in the backyard. It's a world away from the two-bedroom, one bath apartment I grew up in in the Bronx. On the surface, our family looks more or less like the other Fairfield folks: friendly, fit, courteous. But inside I've retained my Bronx roots: straight-talking, tough and skeptical. I know that the grass is greener over here, partly because there *is* grass and lots of it, with manicured lawns and "people" who arrive weekly to care for them. I have "people" too.

When I was young, I remember reading descriptions of spring where the air smelled like perfume. But I doubted the smell of flowers could really overtake bus-exhaust fumes. For me, as the weather got warmer, the stench of the garbage increased outside our building. When I was a little girl, I once smelled a rose on a fence by a private home some blocks from my apartment building, and the scent was faint but beautiful. But you'd need a lot of flowers to cover up the smell of a busy city street in the Bronx.

These days, I live on an officially declared "Scenic Road." Across the street is a farm with a barn from 1790 that still stands. Some trees are clearly as old as the 1830's houses they surround. Horses graze in the fields around many homes in my neighborhood. Stone walls, just like in the Peter Rabbit story books, separate each property and are a backdrop to foxgloves, tiger day lilies and dogwood trees. Now on spring days, I drive home with the sunroof open and realize it's true: After a long hard winter, magnolia trees, the golden forsythia bushes, the colorful tulips and the grass growing greener serve as nature's air freshener. Inevitably, I take a deep breath and feel such gratitude for how far I've come.

As Gary belts in, I feel a similar sense of gratitude. I appreciate that I can afford to take him to Wild Rice, his favorite Japanese restaurant. Growing up, my mom found going out to lunch "too extravagant." If we did buy lunch, we'd go to Lieberman's deli for a grilled hot dog with mustard and sauerkraut and greasy fries to go. We'd eat them while watching soap operas in front of the TV at home. I preferred not eating in public with my mom. Like many teens, I was embarrassed; I wanted to be with the cool kids. Part of my excitement of lunch with Gary is that he is still willing to be seen in public with me. (Or he is just willing to be seen with me because the trade-off of Japanese lunch is worth it.) No matter. As Gary opens the door to Wild Rice for me, the waiter stands by the entrance holding two menus and says hello. We ate here last week and probably the week before. He seats us at our favorite table by the window.

"The regular?" he says, with a warm smile. "I know, no seeds." The waiter knows about Gary's disease because Gary told him. This candor is a consistent trait in Gary's personality and it seems to serve him well. The fact that even the waiter knows not to serve him seeds proves Gary is becoming a self-advocate. He is growing up. I am so proud of him.

Gary gives a wide smile and a nod back. Gary's smile lights up my heart. For three years now he's had Crohn's disease, a chronic digestive disorder that can send him to the bathroom 20 times a day with abdominal cramps that double him over in pain. At first, to attempt to reduce his symptoms, he'd barely eat. With so little nutrition in his body, exhaustion was a daily obstacle. Now, he's learned how to keep the Crohn's in check by eating right. He can make it through the school day, play on the tennis team, be active in activities – and not even need a nap.

Gary picks up his chopsticks and nibbles on the pickled carrots and gingered cabbage on the table. I blurt out, "How was the test?"

"Fine," he says.

It is the typical teenager monosyllabic response and it drives me crazy. It's not like we have to talk only during a commercial break, like I did with my mom. I want details! But I decide not to push too hard, yet. So I ask about something he is excited about. "What's going on with the money for the water pump for South Africa?"

"It is really tough, Mom," he mumbles. So much for my hopes of generating enthusiasm. "The kids in the club have a lot of fundraiser ideas. But we need $14,000. That is a lot of bake sales." He looks up at me like I might have an answer. I don't. I pick up my chopsticks and munch on some carrots as well. Looking out the window of the restaurant, I remember the last time I tried to get my hands on some money.

Three years ago, around the same time we learned about Gary's Crohn's diagnosis, my husband, Steve, was laid off as a hospital administrator. We scoured our budget and eliminated expenses. Easy hits included: no more extended cable channels, no home newspaper delivery, no more phone line with the dedicated fax machine. The small dollars really added up. To make ends meet I worked triple hard growing my young business selling long-term care insurance.

Still, I wondered how we could maintain the same lifestyle and manage financially. I remember sitting on our deck, worried. I was fretting about not being able to send my two sons to camp the following summer as well as the other financial changes we'd need to make. I watched Gary search for frogs in our backyard wetlands, his favorite pastime. Suddenly, my Bronx roots kicked in. My childhood taught me to adapt to circumstances. I grew up playing handball, not tennis. I learned to ride a bike in a crowded parking lot, not on a cul-de-sac. By age 10, if I wanted to go to a movie, I'd take the city bus, by myself.

In Fairfield, we haven't tried to keep up with everyone. My kids have learned to find joy in simple things, like spending hours exploring the woods by our house. *It's not what you have, but what you do that counts*. I have said this in our house at least a thousand times. Gary and his younger brother, Matt, roll their eyes because they've heard it so many times.

When Gary was in elementary school, he'd come bursting through the front door, exclaiming, "Tony got a Wii!"

"It's not what you have, but what you do that counts."

Or, "Sam has a car with a real motor in it!"

"It's not what you have, but what you do that counts."

"Tim's parents put in a pool and a batting cage!"

"It's not what you have, but what you do that counts."

Gary and Matt stopped asking for things.

Fortunately, our kids found activities they could do for free. Gary liked catching frogs. As I sat on the deck pondering about camp, I glanced down at the September Family Circle magazine and saw an article about a contest sponsored by National Geographic Kids. They were looking for the next generation of explorers. The winners would go to South Africa on an expedition the following summer to see "the big five" land animals: lions, elephants, leopards, rhinos and cape buffalos. The air was crisp and cool as I read the contest rules. Winning the contest would solve the camp problem, at least for one child.

I yelled down, "Gary, you want to enter a contest?"

I knew he wouldn't automatically say no, because that is another thing I've drilled into their heads: "Don't close a door before it is opened." Gary would roll his eyes at that one too but I ignored him because my father drilled this into me and I knew I was sitting on my deck overlooking my pool, garden and frog pond because I'd pursued every opportunity open to me.

"What do I have to do?" Gary screamed back.

"Take a picture and write an essay about your favorite place to explore." I knew it sounded like work so I continued, "You could go to South Africa and see real lions!"

"Really? Cool," he said as he descended off a tree trunk and started walking toward the deck.

"Will it take long?" he said with some hesitation in his voice.

"Well, you can go watch TV for a couple of hours – or you can just take a picture of our wetlands and tell them how much you like it." I tried to sound super enthusiastic. I'd read the small print that said the winner could take a parent along on the trip. I'd always wanted to go on safari and the reality was that Steve and I could not afford it.

Gary didn't miss a beat. "Mom, would you get the camera please? I'll tell them about the frogs."

I snap right out of my daydream as the waiter puts Gary's bento box on the table. Sesame seeds are sprinkled on top of the chicken and on the outside of the California roll.

"No seeds!" I scream, my Bronx roots trumping my Connecticut etiquette. Because of the Crohn's, Gary's intestines are inflamed; these seeds could get stuck, and then Gary will be mired in massive pain for the rest of the day. One seed and he won't be able to stand up straight. The experience sounds similar to having a massive kidney stone. He is miserable until it passes.

"Mom, you are embarrassing me," Gary whispers. His quiet to my loudness confirms we clearly were raised in two very different environments.

"Look, you can't have seeds." I don't lower my voice one notch. The waiter knew the expectation. He failed. That is not delivering quality service. From my GE corporate days, when I was an engineer working on the Stealth fighter, it's been drilled into me that quality is meeting the expectation of the customer.

The waiter apologizes and brings a second small plate of pickled veggies to munch on until the kitchen remakes the dish. I am disappointed that my hungry, skinny son has to wait longer for his lunch and I have to wait longer to find out about the PSAT. Instead of talking, we wait for our food in silence. I do not have an answer for Gary about raising money for the water pump. I do not have lunch. So, I make myself look out the window and remember that contest again.

Gary loves animals. He volunteers every week at our local Audubon, down the street, caring for little animals like raptors, lizards and snakes. Gary loves feeding frozen mice to the raptors. I grew up killing roaches in the bathroom and avoiding rats in the incinerator room. I could have provided the Audubon with an unlimited supply of rodents for free! I think the rodents are gross. But Gary's passion may get me on a Safari. On the deck that day I raced to get the camera for a shot of a frog, tossing around the clutter in the closet. My mom, who was resting in the den, heard me making a racket.

"What is going on?" she shrieked in her annoyed voice. When things seem chaotic she gets nervous so she covers it up with New York bravado and just screams. I didn't quite answer quickly enough so she yelled louder. "WHAT. IS. GOING. ON?"

My mom is 81 years old and lives with us. This was our long-term care plan, to all live together in Connecticut. It was a win-win scenario. My parents would care for my children as I held down my big executive job at GE and my husband ran an outpatient surgery center. This way my parents could finally move out of the Bronx. My husband and I could take my parents to doctors' appointments and cataract surgeries here and we wouldn't have to worry about them being mugged while they walked to the store.

"Gary wants to enter a contest and he needs a picture of a frog," I told my mother, as if it were obvious.

I grabbed the camera and went to find Gary.

"Here is the camera. Find a frog and snap a picture." I sounded like a drill sergeant.

He climbed up a couple of feet to where the trunk of a tree had broken off. He slowly descended out into the middle of the pond. The pond was covered in algae. To me it was totally disgusting. But the frogs tend to hang out near the part of the tree in the water. Gary knew this and he scurried down the trunk to almost the water's edge.

I yelled, "Get it?"

Before he could answer he slipped. I saw him protect the camera the same way he learned to protect a football when tackled. He landed smack down on the tree. The thud was loud. I wished he'd had on his football gear. But he stood right up and shook himself off, something I think all those football games taught him. His boot was covered in the green yuck. Instead of asking if he was OK, I shouted, "Try again!" Was I so determined for free summer camp that I wasn't even worried about him hurting himself?

"Mom, I need a net. Let's go to the Audubon and get one," he dictated. He was finding solutions and not giving up. I thought to myself, "That's my boy!"

"Great. I'll drive," I said. We raced to the Audubon, which was a minute or two by car from our house. When we arrived, Gary sprinted to the animal room and told his boss how he needed a picture of a frog for a contest.

"Well, it is sunny today but it's been cold. It will be hard to find one," she said. She knew it was probably too late in the season but she didn't want to burst his enthusiasm − or mine.

Gary and I returned to the woods, looking for frogs by the pond. He balanced on fallen tree limbs to get to the water, stood quietly and patiently waiting to hear a deep bull sound, but we heard none. We spent hours but he didn't give up. As the sun started to set, my cellphone rang.

"Where are you?" my mom demanded.

"At the pond," I murmured. It's like I was a child again. We didn't have cellphones when I was young so I was able to escape more easily. I just had to be home by dark. Now, the sun was a big ball of orange hanging just over the horizon. It was not dark yet; we had at least another 20 minutes. But she had a phone. Gary and I left, without a frog. It wasn't worth aggravating her − that would be harder than losing the contest.

When we arrived home my mother was standing at the front double door waving a green and white plastic turtle.

"Look, take the picture of this. They'll never know," she said, using the familiar drill-sergeant tone that I'd picked up. With a statement like that there was no doubt my mom was a city girl too. National Geographic wouldn't be able to tell the difference between a toy plastic turtle and a real frog? We couldn't just give in and take a picture of the toy to make her happy. (Something I typically would do, even as an adult.) Not this time though. I really wanted Gary to win that safari.

Before I said anything, Gary burst out with, "Are you kidding, Grandma?" He just exploded in laughter. I'd never done that − laughed in her face. I never had the guts. But he wasn't being disrespectful. He saw her as funny. I wish I found the humor in her when I was growing up. With Gary holding onto his sides as he laughed so loud, she burst out in laughter as well. I looked at both of them − her with the plastic turtle, him with the net − and broke out in giggles.

We really are like a sit-com family, I realized. I take her too seriously. Earlier in the day, I was fixated on our finances and now we were sharing belly laughs.

Gary spent the evening sitting at the computer and writing about how we don't get bitten by mosquitoes because we live by a pond overpopulated with frogs. It's like New York City in there, crowded with dwellers. He felt everyone should just get frogs and toads instead of bug zappers to kill mosquitoes. The balance of nature became his essay. For a 12-year-old, it was pretty good, I thought to myself, maybe even a winner. Once he revised it.

The next morning, we gave up on the frog search and instead I snapped a picture of Gary, dressed in an orange T-shirt, tan cargo pants and high green water boots back in our pond. He looked like an explorer, holding that net from the Audubon on the tree stump in the water. It was a perfect picture. I rarely take a good shot. Yet, here was Gary, centered perfectly between the net on one side and a wisp of a tall piece of grass next to his cheek on the other. Not even a shadow was miscast. Instead, the light shone perfectly on his body, his cheeks rosy, his light brown hair highlighted. It looked like a picture in one of the National Geographic magazines! He looked like the next generation of explorer. When I viewed the picture right after taking it, I had this feeling it was a winner. I felt I'd had help with the picture, even though I was alone. It was too perfect and too easy. It felt eerie. I had this urge to look up to the sky and just say thank you – to my late father, to God, to the universe – to them all.

With over 5,000 entrants to the National Geographic Kids contest Gary made it beyond round one with his essay and picture. Round two reduced the pool to only 50 contestants. Each were to be interviewed by phone by the National Geographic Kids team. In between finding out that he made it past round one and before round two, Gary was growing skinnier and skinnier. He'd lost the glow in his cheeks that was so predominant in the picture, and he was constantly tired. Gary had had Crohn's less than a year and was struggling to get into remission. He was growing weaker and weaker. The Crohn's expelled out all his nutrition. He barely made it through a day of school. He'd come home, do his homework and fall asleep by 7 p.m.

The only positive thing happening at this time of his life was the possibility of going to South Africa. All he needed was to blow them away on the phone interview. As a marketing executive with TV, radio and print experience under my belt, I gave Gary a big dose of media training. When the National Geographic Kids interview happened he was prepared. He won!

The doctors cleared him to travel to South Africa as long as he'd stay away from seeds and would take his medicine, 12 Pentasa pills a day and two iron supplements. If Crohn's was not going to stop Gary from taking the trip neither was I.

We went together. We observed the animals plus much much more − the hardship of the South Africans in the townships. It changed our lives.

Remembering this story doesn't give me any inkling of how Gary is going to get the money for the water pump. It just makes me feel worse. I just tell him, "You'll find a way."

Gary doesn't look up at me because the waiter arrives with his food. Before the waiter even puts down the bento box, he announces, "No seeds."

I have my regular sushi lunch with five pieces of fish, yellowtail my favorite and a tuna roll, served inside out with sesame seeds. Gary likes that I continue to eat the way I like and do not modify my diet just because he has Crohn's. Gary, now famished, just eats. He picks up a piece of chicken with his chopsticks and smiles after he swallows. I figure now might be a good time to ask about the PSAT. He must feel the pressure to get into a good college, because of how and where we live. My internal drive came from my parents insisting that I could do better than they did. Steve and I have come pretty far ourselves. After that trip to South Africa, Gary came back determined to help the people there. And he redefined "doing better" to mean "doing more for others."

Gary wants to work as a "doctor without borders" and to figure out how to cure Crohn's. He believes he needs to go to an Ivy League school to do these things. I don't want to squash his drive but I don't believe that college pedigree matters as much as the person aiming for success.

And deep down, I know the Crohn's has slowed down his learning. He's missed quite a bit of school. Before he was diagnosed, sometimes the cramps were so bad he'd just stay home. But Gary doesn't want to give up on his dream and who am I to squelch his ambitions? I bet his story will yield an incredible college essay. Now I just wonder if he has the test-taking abilities.

"The test didn't seem too bad," he says. He sounds confident. I am so thrilled I raise my hand to give him a high five.

He slaps me back. Then he mentions, "Oh, Mom? For the past 10 days or so, it really hurts when I pee."

What You Can Do Now

---

1. *Help your loved one to be honest about their condition with other people when appropriate.*

Our family found that people are more understanding than we'd expected. It was freeing for us and our family to be open about Gary's illness.

2. *During a challenging time, look for something tangible and positive to accomplish.*

Like I did with the contest. It didn't matter the outcome, we had fun entering. Plant a tree, bake cookies for a food pantry, or clean a closet. Find something you both can feel good about.

3. *Be grateful.*

It might not seem like anything is going right, but there is always something, each day, to say thank you for. Find it and acknowledge it.

* * *

Chapter 2

Martian Mom in the E.R

I try not to sound too alarmed. "Oh," leaves my lips but my chopstick falls to the floor. I feel my stomach drop with it. Gary tends to minimize his symptoms, so if he says it hurts, he must be feeling serious pain. This is a new pain. Gary's health is a daily delicate balance. In the last three years, he's changed from a football star, one of the strongest and biggest kids in his class, to someone even the smaller kids tower over. And he is so weak and skinny.

He's taken five trips in an ambulance in six weeks. He'd fall to the ground, with his arms flailing, his legs thrashing and him unresponsive. It looked liked seizures and scared everyone, especially me. Gary has no memory of the episodes. The first time, I got the emergency call from the high school tennis coach to meet the ambulance by the tennis courts. Gary seized during tennis tryouts. As he lay on the court, all the kids stood behind the chain-link fence and stared as he was lifted into the ambulance. I rode along in shock. The other four times, he fell to the floor in school. His eyes rolled to the back of his head, and his body shook with varying high frequency, low amplitude jolts. Someone in panic would call the ambulance, and then call me. I'd drop whatever I was doing, try to keep my composure long enough to drive to the scene and not crack the car. But, as I raced to him, I was incapable of holding back my tears. I'd arrive and an EMT would whisk me into the front seat of the ambulance ready to race again. With the sirens blaring and my fingers clawing onto the armrest, we'd swerve between cars until arriving at the E.R.

Once there, it was the same over and over again: Gary would stay about one hour in the E.R., hooked up to fluids. Slowly the shaking would stop and he'd regain consciousness. He'd feel really tired and remember nothing, except maybe a couple of minutes before falling to the ground. The hospital doctors released him each time, saying he'd had an anxiety attack. Besides an M.R.I., which found nothing, there was no additional testing. He received a diagnosis by the E.R. physicians of stress, along with a standard release form stating the doctor's recommendation to see a psychotherapist and to consider taking anxiety medication. Gary would leave the hospital saying, "It's not anxiety, Mom." He was convinced. I didn't know what to think.

After the third attack, the pressure mounted on me from the school to put him on anxiety medication. The school did not want him to hurt himself, say if he fell off a chair. Also, the other kids were scared. One mother called me to say her son was traumatized by seeing Gary's seizure-like episodes. Her son could not concentrate the rest of the day and did poorly on a math test. Somehow this was my fault. My husband was afraid too. He thought maybe we were in denial and that Gary should try the meds. I lost sleep because I didn't want to fight with my husband who agreed with the doctors but I believed my son when he said that he did not feel anxious. I refused to blindly put him on the medications. But the consensus was that the attacks had to stop and the pills should do the trick. I took Gary out of school and then to one specialist after another. Following appointments with a neurologist, endocrinologist and, yes, a psychotherapist, it seemed Gary was right. They concluded Gary was not having anxiety attacks. The endocrinologist finally figured out the problem: Gary was hypoglycemic. His blood sugar would plunge and he'd fall to the ground. The recommended cure was simple: eat smaller meals more frequently. No pills necessary. Gary learned to eat several meals more a day and the result was immediate: No more ambulance rides. I learned something as well: to listen to the patient and to trust my instincts.

This series of episodes launched the start of the new me, the Mom who questioned too-quick doctor diagnoses followed by pharmaceutical remedies.

Now, the patient had a new symptom. *Oy.*

As we sit in the Japanese restaurant, with bamboo plants and tri-fold sake signs on the wooden tables, Gary sweetly says, "Mom, I really want to relax this weekend. Please don't call the doctor today. I'll be OK." I know this tone, sweet and hopeful. He is starting to learn how to charm to get his way. His broad smile and good looks, inherited from his 6'2", green-eyed dad, have him destined to be another Oster lady-killer.

He takes the last bite of the California roll and gives me that smile that makes me melt. I love seeing him happy and inside I hope he is right that he'll be OK.

I say, "Let's see how it goes."

The minute we arrive home after running some errands, Gary runs right to the bathroom. He shouts through the door, "It still hurts to urinate!"

I can tell he underplays the symptom, though, because he does not leave the bathroom for 20 minutes. While he is still in there, I call the doctor's office. It's after 5 p.m. on Saturday and a tired-sounding nurse answers the phone. "We are closing up for the day. The answering line should have picked up. Is this a medical emergency?"

"I'm not sure," I tell her. "It hurts my son to urinate. He is 15 years old." I know that age is the first question they ask, so I just include it in my response.

"Well, have him drink some cranberry juice and call back in the morning. On Sunday we open at 8:30. Just be aware, with the swine flu season underway, I suggest you call early to get an appointment."

I work full time selling insurance to people and I really like to sleep in on Sundays. To occupy the kids, Steve takes Gary and Matt to Super Stop & Shop for the weekly grocery shopping order. Our family's survival method for our pressure-filled work life is a steady routine at home. By food shopping early Sunday morning, we are prepared if our work requirements create chaos when we least expect it. This way, there is always milk in the fridge for the boys. My guys are out of the house by 7 a.m. My kids are like their dad, early risers. Steve really seems to relish this male bonding time together. With our hectic lives, it's the one time every week Steve can be alone with them. He tells me how the kids race through the store and buy their favorite foods for the week, all while sipping Dunkin' Donuts hot chocolate and munching on bagels. Once home, they rush to put all the groceries away and tell me the surprise they bought for me to cook for our Sunday night family dinner.

They creep out of the house for the store thinking I am asleep. I am frantic to get through to the doctor's office. It still hurts Gary to pee. He didn't elaborate too much but he said it's been 10 days. So, it doesn't seem to be going away on its own. By 8 a.m. my fingers are punching the buttons on the phone. The line is already busy. Swine flu must be sweeping Connecticut just as the nurse reports. I love the redial button. I hear the deep toned Beep Beep Beep, hang up and hit the redial button, hard, over and over again. Finally at 8:35, I hear a voice on the line and am told to have him in the office by 9. I can't believe they want to see him so quickly. Even though Gary is not home from the market yet, I take the appointment. I know the routine: My husband and kids should be walking in the door any second. Just as I hang up the phone, I hear the garage door opening up. Our dog, Chloe, a loveable black and brown mutt, barks on cue. In our family, even the dog is predictable. As Gary carries two bags of groceries into the kitchen, I tell him we have to leave for the doctor's office immediately.

"Mom, can't I make scrambled eggs first? I'm starved." I know he ate bagels in Stop & Shop and he probably wants to avoid going to the doctor.

"Nope. We got to go," I say. I'm very concerned but don't want him to know. I reach for the car keys on the kitchen counter top and dash to the garage where I see Steve picking up more bags of groceries. Steve looks tired, but not from lack of sleep, more from concern about Gary. Steve's hair is almost completely gray now. Without saying anything to each other, I know we are both concerned.

"Doctor wants to see him. Now." I say *now* with the emphasis that sums up our distress. "I'll call you to keep you posted." I tenderly kiss Steve's lips. I turn on the engine as Gary strolls into the garage.

October on our country lane is especially beautiful. The morning sun illuminates the red barn across the street and the horses seem to bask in its rays to warm their bodies from the chilly night. Their calm is a stark contrast to my heart palpitations. The doctor wants to see him so fast? Ten days of pain? Hurts to urinate? What is going on? I hate being late and I know it only takes 10 minutes on back roads to get to the doctor's office, so I try to calm myself down by watching the horses. Maybe some of their peacefulness can rub off on me. Gary remarks about the orange color of the old oak tree on the corner across from the 1830's house.

"It's like a big pumpkin," he says, sounding like he really doesn't want to talk about his symptoms and beating me to break the silence, because I'd just bring up the Crohn's.

I say, "You know, it's Grandma's favorite season. I bet she'd love to see this tree."

He declares, "I'll show it to her later, when we get back."

He sounds determined that he'll be home to watch football later with his Dad. He picks up his iPod and inserts the ear pieces for the rest of the ride. I keep thinking about his future. Most sophomores are not racing to the doctor today. They are doing school work or playing sports. They are doing what is needed to get into college.

Gary is brought into an examining room by a nurse. No wait? Gary's pediatrician, Lisa Miller, M.D., a petite Ivy League graduate with a quick smile, teenagers of her own and an aura of quiet confidence, enters seconds later. I like her because she is a mom, too. She understands my concern without saying anything. She gets right down to business and asks only questions about Gary's health. She seems to push on his stomach in a prescribed way. It's like she already knows what is going on, even though see can't see underneath his skin. She feels her way.

"Ow," he says, wincing but trying to be a cool teenager without any drama.

She turns to me, "I'd like you to consider taking him to the emergency room in Norwalk. I can't run tests here. They can run an ultrasound." I'm thinking this doesn't sound good but I don't want to let my fright show. I don't want to scare Gary.

"Oh," I say, dreading another trip to the E.R. but grateful it is a Sunday and it's Norwalk; it's quieter and quicker on Sundays in the Norwalk E.R. The worst is Saturday night in the Bridgeport Hospital E.R. Bridgeport is a tough town, typically with a lot of trauma on a weekend night. When Gary went to the E.R. there one Saturday night, so many patients had critical knife and gunshot wounds that the doctors left Gary to seize on a gurney in the hall. I just stood clinging onto the gurney until Gary stopped seizing and fell asleep. Another time, a PCP addict was chained down on a gurney with the policeman at the criminal's side, right next to Gary. The police officer stood so close to Gary, I think Gary could have reached out and touched the officer's gun. The policeman bragged that it took three taser zaps to get the big brawny bad guy down. Now, the prisoner was screaming profanities. "Fuck this life! Fuck you." When Gary came to, he heard the racket and saw the cops.

"See what drug use does?" the officer warned, leaning in to Gary's face. It was an education many kids don't get and I wish mine had missed as well.

By Sunday morning most of the hoodlum stuff is probably already over. We should be fine in Norwalk.

"We know that emergency room. We've been there before during one of his seizure attacks," I tell the doctor. I turn to Gary and say, "Are you OK with going? This will be a first – you won't arrive in an ambulance. I'll drive you." I was trying to make it sound positive.

"Yeah, let's go. I'll see what it is like when I am conscious." Clearly he was responding to my upbeat attitude.

It is not even 10 a.m. as we pull in to the E.R. As I'd hoped, it's quiet here. Busy or quiet, the process is the same as always. The admitting nurse asks his name and looks it up. She sees Gary's record in the system, a reality, I think to myself, I wish were someone else's. I am becoming used to the E.R. and can't believe this process is part of my life. I hand over my insurance card before she even asks.

He's put in bay 27, a small room with essential emergency equipment. I hear on the overhead sound system Gloria Gaynor's "I Will Survive," a personal favorite of mine from my dating years' sagas. I think to myself, how many times did that song give me strength? A broken heart used to seem like the end of the world. Now, it feels like a feather compared to the lead weight of not knowing why my son is in such pain. I vow to myself, I will survive and I will help him survive. As we get settled in the room, I hear the nurses say they'll be listening to 70's music all day.

Gary asks to go to the bathroom. Now that he's admitted it hurts, he must feel free to scream in the bathroom. He sounds like the convict: "Fuck this!" It takes about 20 minutes for the pain to subside. When he returns I don't comment about his language. My heart breaks to see such a normal function be so hard for him. He tells me he just wants someone to tell him that he is not nuts, that the pain is real and something is causing it. I hold his hand as he sits on the gurney waiting for the doctor.

Dr. Greenberg, a 40-ish doctor with broad shoulders and a fast handshake, enters Gary's station. He presses on Gary's stomach, the same exact way Dr. Miller did earlier, and says that they need to do a CT scan. I dutifully ask all the questions about radiation risk. But I sense there really is not a choice. It is the start of what I have now come to think of as the protocol train, a journey that follows a prescribed track without necessarily knowing the trip's destination.

At this point on the track, Dr. Greenberg sounds like a robot as he answers my questions about radiation. He's been on this part of the ride many times before. His answers are fact-based with disclosures about potential risk. He tells me the pros outweigh the cons. He needs to know what is going on inside Gary. The doctor seems to be moving Gary like he's freight following a scheduled route. As I listen, I realize the train needs to follow this track to move forward.

"He'll have to drink liquid contrast and wait a couple of hours for the liquid to go through his system so I can see his intestines on the CT scan," the doctor states. The doctor's tone bothers me but his confidence seems to set Gary's mind at ease.

Gary knows he probably won't have to urinate again for hours and, his pain temporarily gone, he asks for my cellphone. He calls Steve and asks him to bring his backpack to the emergency room so he can do his bio homework. Inside I am proud of him because he wants to stay on his college track. Within the hour Steve delivers the backpack. The liquid for Gary to drink looks gross, but not as bad as the barium they use to make the lower bowel more visible. Gary had to suffer through that when he was first diagnosed. The taste of the barium, used to diagnose the Crohn's, was horrible and it was torture for him to drink the stuff. Steve repeats the counting games they used the first time to get him to drink the barium. "Beat me with a gulp by the time I count to four." Then Steve counts so fast, it seems impossible. But Gary still tries. So, Steve counts again real fast. Gary tries again. It's so impossible that Gary breaks out in laughter and almost spits out the stuff.

"Remember the barium, Dad, from the first time? This stuff is not as bad as that." Before he takes a swig, he recites, "This isn't barium and I don't have to pee." He says it like he knows things really could be worse. This time he empties the Styrofoam cup more easily. Once he gets down the final swig of liquid, Gary tells his dad to go home. "Go rest. I'll be fine. Mom will call you with the results," he says.

I am proud of how he handles this new crisis. Instead of wanting to be babied, Gary seems more concerned for his dad. Just last year, my husband was laid off again from his job and had his own scary medical crisis that required surgery. The importance of health insurance became very clear to our family. Gary and Steve both have pre-existing medical conditions now so health insurance is very expensive for us. To get our family coverage when Steve was unemployed, we were paying approximately $1,800 a month! With jobs scarce, Steve swallowed his pride and took a new job at half his former pay but with full medical benefits. Many friends told Steve to keep looking because he was worth more. But Steve and I decided to further cut back our expenses and take the job. Little did we know how good of a decision this would be. Gary witnessed first-hand how important a job is beyond just the pay. Steve's job was our best way to get health insurance at a reasonable price.

To be productive on the job, Steve needs to stay healthy. So Gary knows his dad still needs to rest. He also knows his grandmother, who gets crazy with worry, will need calming down. After all, her grandson is in the E.R.! So, Gary kisses his dad again and says, "I'll be fine. Go home. Take care of my little bro and Grandma. They need you at home. Mom's here."

I wish Steve could stay with me. I think if Gary didn't act so brave, I would have told Steve to stay even though he needs the weekend to rejuvenate himself by resting. I feel weak in my knees just waiting to find out the source of Gary's pain. I take a deep breath as I walk behind Gary on the stretcher to the CT machine. The halls leading to the CT scan machine are familiar to me. Gary had an M.R.I. of his brain here after his first "seizure-like" episode. With all the hospital visits under my belt, I know the most important thing for me is to be strong for Gary. I force myself to stay steady. Carrying on with emotional dramatics before any information is a waste of my energy and only scares him. This could turn out to be nothing or an easy fix.

As they close the doors for the CT scan, they shoo me outside to reduce my exposure to radiation. Gary is wheeled alone into the room. I stand under the florescent lights on linoleum floor feeling as stark as my surroundings. The only things breaking the monotony of the long corridor are a wooden side table against a wall and some Home Style magazines next to a chair. I sit down and try to take my mind off my reality by reading. Truth is I can't read a word. I thumb through the pages to look like I am reading. Actually, I just pray. My thoughts are interrupted by an attendant wheeling Gary out of the room.

"All done. You should have the results in 20 minutes," the attendant says as she wheels Gary back to the E.R.

This reminds me of when I wait for a picture from the rollercoaster ride at Six Flags Amusement Park, the picture at the biggest drop, the one that captures my fear. It appears at the counter for purchase. I never buy it.

Gary is wheeled back to bay 27 and our waiting begins. Gary pulls out his bio homework and puts his notebook on a cart. To hide the tears welling up in me I find focusing on his homework helps. He draws a plant cell where he colors the ribosome red and the mitochondria green. He clearly identifies all the parts and reads the text book to answer the questions on the worksheet. Gary even has time to finish his Latin homework.

So much for the 20-minute wait. Probably an hour passes and we start to hear the doctors talking. I peek out of the curtain and try to hear what they're saying. Dr. Greenberg, on the phone, is hidden behind a computer screen. He can't see me and probably thinks I am not as close as I am to him. In the background, I hear Simon and Garfunkel singing *Bridge Over Troubled Water*. The words describe me to a "T." I am weary. I am feeling small and I need another tissue to wipe away my tears. Waiting for results is the worst part. I feel so alone. Where is the bridge? I turn around to try to hear the doctors' conversation over the music. With all the medical speak, the only words I clearly hear and understand are, "mass next to the bladder."

I shudder.

"Mom, can you hear anything?"

"They see something. So it's not your imagination." I can't tell him what I think I hear. I'm terrified. My tears start to flow. I pretend to sneeze so I have a reason for grabbing a tissue from my handbag.

"I'm glad because I know it hurts. It *has* to be something. This isn't my imagination." He sounds happy that he is not crazy.

I am sure I am like every other mom to think that "mass" means tumor and tumor means cancer. That's what it meant with my father. My fear is something I do not share with Gary. I take a deep breath and walk to get a cup for some water. As the cold water fills the cup, I hear the Bee Gees sing "Stayin' Alive." Barry Gibbs sings it at the top of his lungs in perfect pitch. I walk back to Gary's gurney and quietly harmonize, "You're staying alive." I'm used to having to be the strong one, but even my mental antics to think positive are not fooling me. I don't let Gary see my knees wobble. I softly ask, "When should we call Dad?" I give him the option, so he feels some control.

"Wait till we hear from the doctor. No need to worry Grandma," he says.

I wish my mother would comfort me and not vice versa, especially now. My mother is a heavyset, vocal, New York City native, who tends toward emotional hysteria. I'd like to say it's her age but she's always been this way. She thinks screaming is talking and yells even when faced with a problem the size of a molehill. Gary knows this. Possible tumor, this is Everest. I can't imagine how loud she'd scream if I told her.

Last year when Steve was unemployed, I needed to support the family. In long-term-care insurance sales I have control over my hours because I set my own appointments. Unlike my highly compensated GE job, which I left after 18 years, this is a 100 percent commission-based business. The more I sell the more money I make. The business is a perfect fit for a family because I have control over my hours and my income. Plus, I have time to always take my mom for her doctor appointments, to the hair-dresser or on errands.

When Steve was unemployed and not feeling well, his doctor wanted him to have a brain scan to check for a possible brain tumor. On the morning that Steve went to the doctor for the scan, I wanted to go with him but I had a big deal to close. We needed the money and we both went our separate ways. My mom stayed home alone where her thoughts could race and race. That afternoon, when I came home between appointments, my mom's pulse was at 130 and it would not go down. She couldn't stand up, her color was gray. She was sitting in the living room, a place mostly for looking at, not using, because it's filled with her furniture from her apartment. It's the good stuff.

"I'm fine," she panted as she sat breathless on the living room chair. "Take care of Steve."

Pulse racing, heart pounding. She needed medical attention, stat. Was this a heart attack? A stroke? I was clueless and terrified. This mountain felt too big for me. Steve was still at the doctor having his brain scanned. She refused for me to call an ambulance for her, but agreed to let me drive her to urgent care where the doctor immediately put her in an ambulance. With sirens blazing, I followed the ambulance to Bridgeport Hospital. As I carefully drove behind the ambulance, my cellphone rang with a disgruntled client on the other end. My client screamed at me about a billing mistake the insurance carrier had made. I needed to be at my computer to answer her question, but I listened and let her complain. She calmed down. Inside I wanted to scream that her problem was nothing compared to mine at the moment. But I needed the money. I did not want her to cancel her insurance.

As I pulled into the E.R. parking lot I finally said, "The siren you heard is the ambulance with my mother in it. She may be having a heart attack. I just arrived in the parking lot. I hope you'll understand that I'll have to call you back later."

"Oh my God, Randi, go to your mom. Don't worry about me. We'll speak later in the week. Thanks for listening. Now go."

Luckily the client was a nurse. She never did cancel the insurance.

I sprinted to the E.R. and found my mom on a gurney. The doctor gave her a drug which instantly slowed her heart down. He said she was having a panic attack, not a heart attack. He asked her what happened. In a New York minute, she explained, "Well, doctor, my son-in-law lost his job and is sick. He might lose his medical insurance. Today, he went to see if he has a brain tumor. My grandson has Crohn's disease and his medications are expensive." She said this with the drama of an Academy Award-winning actress, although the reality did not take much acting. It was a real mountain this time.

"Ah, I get it," said the doctor, who looked as if he'd only recently started shaving. "That can make anyone anxious." Then he looked at me.

"So, this is your mother and she is concerned about your unemployed husband who might have a brain tumor, and your son is sick with Crohn's?"

"Yes," I said. He'd summed it up pretty well.

"So, how are you doing?" He looked directly at me.

Wait, let's pause on this. Someone actually asked me about me. I was floored. I was so used to meeting everyone else's needs to help them with their lives that I didn't think about my needs. I smiled, and maybe gave off some nervous laughter.

"Doctor, I am fine. I have to be. I need to support this family," I said with the confidence of a high wire performer.

He looked at me like I was a Martian because I was too calm, too together. I was the opposite of my mother, probably the opposite of many loved ones with someone in the E.R. I don't know, but he looked at me with curiosity. What he didn't understand was that even though I was scared to my core, I accepted that these problems were beyond my abilities to solve, alone. I couldn't take away my son's Crohn's, my husband's possible brain tumor, my Mom's process for dealing (or not dealing) with anxiety. All I could do was to try to help everyone get better. I prayed to God that if he'd take care of the future, I'd work on the present. It was my only hope. If I got through the day, I knew the future would be here soon enough. This way I didn't have to worry about tomorrow, just make today as good as possible. Instead of telling the doctor this explanation, which might seem too spiritual, I shared the "laughter is the best medicine" approach.

"Someone once told me this trick," I said. "When bad things happen, pretend you see elephants, like Dumbo, flying around your head. When something bad happens, visualize the elephants pooping on your head." He looked at me even more quizzically.

I just continued. "Imagine it like a cartoon episode. You know how the coyote always gets blown up chasing the road runner? It's hysterical."

"OK, flying pooping elephants, like Dumbo. How does this help you?" The sincerity in his voice hinted that he was dealing with some problems of his own.

"I just focus on cleaning up each poop. Some poops are bigger than others. Sometimes the elephants poop and they miss. Like my mom didn't have a heart attack. Now, I can even laugh at the elephants for screwing up. They didn't get me or her. It's not as bad as it could have been. I'll just take her home to rest. I am grateful. You see, if I take care of one poop at a time, I end up with a clean floor instead of standing in dung." I reached for my mother's hand and she just smiled at the doctor.

My mom said, "See, the elephants missed." She even laughed.

He signed her release papers as he said, "Thank you." He looked me in the eye.

"For what?" I asked, as I grabbed the cane for my mother.

"For showing me how to handle the poop. The elephants poop a lot around me and whether it's a direct hit or not, I tend to get aggravated. My wife will love to see me laugh more as I handle typical shit." He spoke right from his heart, not one iota of pretense.

My daydream is interrupted by Dr. Greenberg entering. He sits down on the chair next to Gary's gurney. A guy who identifies himself as the general surgeon stands next to the bed. They both are graying men in their late 40's, maybe even early 50's. They are in good shape with pleasant demeanors. I automatically assume their lives are easier than mine, and, with their years of experience, they probably know how to handle elephant poop, too.

"This case is not for me," the general surgeon announces.

"Oh?" I feel relieved.

"I am not a pediatric surgeon and this has to with his bladder. He needs a urologist," he says and starts walking to the computer. "If you want I can show you the scan on the computer."

Here comes the rollercoaster picture. I feel my knees buckle as I walk toward the screen. Gary is already two steps ahead of me. He can't wait to see the shot. Gary thrives on watching medical surgical shows on TV. His favorite program is "Untold Stories of the E.R." I cringe when I see blood oozing from wounds and surgeons cutting open skin. Gary watches their technique for operating, hoping one day he'll be that surgeon. Gary walks to the computer monitor in the center of the E.R. Dr. Greenberg stands in front of the P.C. He starts scrolling through the images of Gary's internal organs. It's sort of like seeing an ultrasound of a baby. You sort of can see the outline but it really looks like a bad ink blot.

"See that?" the doctor says, sounding excited. "Your bladder should be round and yours is kidney shaped. It's because of this mass next to it."

There is that dreaded word again and the doctor just blurts it out! This is his bedside manner? Who trained this guy? Without flinching or showing any emotion, I look for a reaction from Gary. As my pressure builds inside, I think I feel a few more gray hairs pop out.

"I see it, Doctor." Gary says this with an air of excitement. I don't think he knows the correlation between mass and tumor.

Anyway, this confirms that the pain is not his imagination.

"You have a leak from your bladder and this formed an abscess and bacteria got caught in it. Your body healed a wall around the abscess to protect itself and this wall is pushing on your bladder. That is why it hurts to urinate. We spoke to your gastroenterologist, Dr. Simmon, and he wants you to start on an antibiotic right away. That should kill the infection. He wants you to call him in the morning for a face-to-face check-up."

"It's an infection, Doctor, and it's liquid in the mass?" I gently ask, anxiously waiting for a reply.

"Yes, the antibiotics should do the trick," he states.

I am ecstatic. It's not cancer? It's something antibiotics can kill off? I've been scared, queasy and thrilled all while confined to this place. As Gary puts on his shoes to leave, I hear the O'Jays singing on the sound system, encouraging me to join the love train. Turns out, it is not a rollercoaster but a *Love Train*.

After seven hours in the emergency room and a prescription for two antibiotics, Gary says, "I'm starved, Mom, can you make the steak we bought this morning for dinner?"

I say yes at the speed of a high speed locomotive.

I am so glad to be leaving this station, but deep down I suspect the ride is not over.

What You Can Do Now

---

1. Trust your instincts and your loved one's instincts.

Ask questions. If you are still uncomfortable with the answers, don't give in. Give yourself the time to find an expert who will listen and explain the diagnosis to your satisfaction. When Gary said he did not have anxiety, I believed him. I took him to specialist after specialist to find out what was causing his seizure-like episodes.

2. Hold back your fear in front of your loved one, until you have a diagnosis.

For me, waiting for the diagnosis is the worst part. But, the results may not be as bad as you fear. Your loved one feeds off your energy. The more positive you are, the more confidence you give him or her. With Gary, I really believed the tumor was cancer. I was so wrong. I am glad to this day that I never bothered him with my personal panic.

3. Complete one action item at a time.

A health crisis is overwhelming. It is easy to let the daily grind slip into the next day's grind. But eventually the to-do pile will be massive. Stay focused on completing one task at a time. Eliminating even a few tasks will take some pressure off you. Even though I was racing behind an ambulance with my mother inside, I still listened to my complaining client. If I hadn't, she would have escalated the issue higher. I resolved the problem and was able to move on to the next action item.

* * *

Chapter 3
A Disease Progressing

I wait for my morning tea to steep. I attempt to read the Connecticut Post. But I am really wondering how Gary fared last night. After that rollercoaster ride, they released him with a prescription for antibiotics. He went to bed right after dinner and never woke me. Yesterday's excitement drained me and I slept soundly. This morning, I gaze at the golden leaves falling from the oak tree outside and I place my hand on the teapot to feel its warmth. It's only when I finally hear the sound of Gary's footsteps that I am brought back to reality.

Before I can even ask how he is, Gary blurts out, "Good morning. Mom, I'm fine. I want to go to school today." He doesn't let me get a word in and continues, "I just won't drink too much." Then he says in a softer tone, "But, can you please drive me? I still have to go to the bathroom and I'll miss the bus."

He's dismayed that he needs me to drive him because it is a reminder that he is not well. When he was first diagnosed with Crohn's and went to the bathroom 20 times a day, I drove him to school often. I don't mind driving him; I'm happy that I have the flexibility to do so. I've told him this over and over again. But I think he really wants to be independent. He remembers my days as an executive in GE; I think they made an indelible mark on him. In those days, we all had to leave early. I didn't want to be a barking drill sergeant mom, so starting in kindergarten, I taught my kids to wake themselves, dress themselves, make breakfast themselves, get their homework packed themselves and leave on time for the bus themselves. Selfishly, I needed them to be responsible for … themselves; keeping my high level position in GE required my full attention. Steve was out of the house earlier than they were, but he tried to be home for dinner. Me too. I remember the stress of those days too well, feeling like I was always in the wrong place. At work, I wanted to be home. At home, I felt I needed to be working. I left that world after my father passed away, when Gary was in third grade. Now, I am in the right place – for my family.

Going to the bathroom seems to take Gary more time than usual this morning. I hear him screaming "fuck" as he urinates. I cringe at the sounds and the words on the other side of the bathroom door and hope the antibiotics kick in fast.

I ask, "Are you sure you want to go to school? I'll be booking an appointment with Dr. Simmon for today anyway."

"Mom, listen, it only hurts to pee and the pain lasts about 20 minutes. By the time we get to school, I'll be fine. Besides, we have no idea what time Dr. Simmon will want to see me. It might not be till after school." That kid's attitude amazes me. Besides, he knows from experience how hard it is to catch up.

I drive him to school and we're both quiet in the car. He listens to his iPod. I welcome the silence. I wonder if antibiotics will do the trick or if Dr. Simmon will tell us that more needs to be done. I seem to learn as I go with Crohn's disease, and I deep down wish there were a road map I could follow.

At the school drop-off line, Gary exits the car and throws his backpack on his shoulder. He winces and holds his groin. My heart aches. As he walks toward the school's double entrance doors, he turns around and shouts back, "Mom, it will be better in a few minutes. Thanks for the ride."

It only takes 15 minutes for me to drive home. By 8 a.m. my fingers are dialing the gastroenterologist's office. According to the E.R. release form, Gary needs to be seen by his G.I. doctor, Dr. Simmon, who diagnosed Gary with Crohn's disease three years ago. Gary trusts him because he took away Gary's pain once before and stopped him from needing to go to the bathroom 20 times a day. Since then, Gary has regular bowel movements, very few cramps and, best from his perspective, has grown at least two inches.

Gary especially likes Dr. Simmon because the doctor understood that Gary did not want to follow medical protocol and take prednisone, a steroid, to reduce the number of bowel movements per day. Dr. Simmon had explained to Gary the side effects of the steroid and how it could give him a round face and possible anxiety. I knew it could also stunt growth. Awful. But if that's what the doctor chose, I'd follow his directions – back then, anyway. Because Gary's symptoms were not considered severe, the doctor presented Gary with an option, a nutritional route, which included not eating anything solid for a whole month and drinking liquid supplements instead. He warned Gary that most kids find nutritional therapy very difficult to stick with. At age 12, though, the round face possibility seemed worse to Gary. He wanted so much to be like everyone else. So, he chose not to eat for a month and to just drink the supplements. It was not easy to do, but for Gary the tradeoff of looking normal was worth it. For maintenance, he took a mild medication, Pentasa, and it seemed to work. Now, Gary totally trusts Dr. Simmon.

I place the call for the appointment and it's too early still. I get the answering service folks who explain to me that offices open up at 8:30 a.m. With a half hour to spare, I check my appointments for the day and have my assistant reschedule clients. Hopefully they will rebook appointments for another day. This is stressing me out, though, because I don't want to lose the potential business. I start dialing the doctor's office at 8:29 a.m. and get a busy signal. Once again, I love the redial button. After yesterday's pounding, I am amazed it still works. The wording is faded but I know which one to hit. I ram the button over and over again with each busy signal. Luckily for me and the phone, I get through at 8:35 a.m. The nurse at the gastroenterologist's office tells me to bring Gary in at 11:30 a.m.

Since the drive from our home to the gastroenterologist's office at Children's Hospital in Hartford takes about an hour and a half, I immediately call the school. The receptionist recognizes my voice, from all the other times she's transferred me to the school nurse, again reinforcing a reality that I wish were someone else's. This time, I ask for the dean, Mr. Sanchez. The school administrators seem a little afraid of Gary. His seizure-like episodes, understandably, scared many students and the staff. Mr. Sanchez once followed the ambulance to the E.R. to check on Gary. He ended up hugging and holding me while Gary lay there, shaking and unconscious.

"Please, Mr. Sanchez, I have to have Gary outside by the student pick-up line by 10 a.m. It's an emergency. I am taking him up to Children's Hospital today." He recognizes my tone and doesn't ask any questions. He just says, "No problem" and hangs up the phone.

"Grandma, get your cane. We're going to pick up Gary at school," I shout out to my mother. I started calling her Grandma when she moved in with us years ago. Otherwise we'd have two people with the same name – "Mom" – living under one roof. Now our names and roles are clear. I've learned, it's less stressful for Grandma to be with us than to be alone wondering and worrying about what is happening. It also gets her out of the house and walking, something her doctor told me she needs. Besides, Grandma loves to treat Gary to lunch at Chowder Pot IV, only minutes from Children's Hospital, after a doctor's appointment. Chowder Pot IV is another of Gary's favorite restaurants. He loves the lobster. We've made it pretty much part of the routine to go after the doctor's appointment. I'll do anything to fatten him up and so will Grandma, including paying for the lobster lunch. I get a salad to try to balance out the cost.

Grandma moves slowly, but this is relatively new. In her prime she was as strong as an ox. Not even chain-smoking and fast food dinners every night slowed her down. She once even got a mugger in the Bronx to cry instead of taking her wallet. She screamed at him, "This will make your mother proud?" Her voice is deep and I still shiver when I hear her yelling for something. Now, she screams, "Where are my eyeglasses?" or "Where is my pocketbook?" The kids race to help her and laugh when the glasses are on her head or her purse is by her feet. It's a comedy show at our house. She laughs too. She also likes order so we keep everything in its place, otherwise she'll scream until she finds a missing item and will expect us to drop everything until it is in her hand. We've all learned to repeat most things and we try not to lose patience when she asks the same questions over and over again. She still sees her main job as running the home, her traditional housewife role, so I've made her in charge of laundry, dishes and beds. She loves this job and it is another way I can balance my work life. Sometimes, she even turns down our beds at night with a chocolate. Every day she feels that she can't leave the house until the dishes are done and the laundry is put away. Why? In her words, "In case I die." She doesn't want to leave me anything extra to do, she says.

Still, it's hard. I know I need to rush to pick up Gary, but I try not to let my frustration with Grandma's slow gait show. If she feels old, she'll feel bad, that will take us even longer. Instead, I help her to the car and close the door for her. Just as I sit down to turn on the engine, she commands, "Stop off at CVS to pick up my prescription on the way to school."

I think she is confused because she thinks we are going to Dr. Simmon for a checkup and a lunch, a typical excursion. So, in her mind, I need to do her errands first. I explain again, "I checked. You have another week of medication left. Just because it is ready, doesn't mean we have to go instantly." But the reality is that I am her personal driver and she worries that if Gary may need me I won't be able to go later for her. She wants her medications now, just in case. She concedes, reluctantly, because Gary has to get to the doctor by 11:30, but she still throws in "When are we going to do my stuff?" I rarely do this, but I ignore her and drive directly to the school. I pull up to the high school precisely at 10 a.m. and see Mr. Sanchez, the dean, running to the car. I am touched by his concern and his action. It is further proof to me that people in the school do care.

"We have a slight problem," he says. "Gary's grade is in the auditorium watching a play about drug abuse and it's pitch black in there. We can't see him."

I leave the car parked in the fire lane with Grandma in it. I sprint to the auditorium. The timeline is tight; I have to be on the road now to make the appointment in time. I get to the 750-seat auditorium and pitch black is right. I can't see anyone's face watching the play. I start going up and down the aisles looking for Gary and make out nothing. Not one face. On stage, I see the kids act out how to say "no" to drugs. Sometimes a scene in the play calls for an actor to be under the spotlight. The light diffuses, slightly illuminating the people in the seats. When the spotlight is on, I can sort of make out the faces of the kids in the rows. It is too hard waiting for a spotlight. Should I have them stop the play and make an announcement? My mom would have done that when I was young. She'd not think how totally embarrassed I'd be. My mom would have created a ruckus. Right now, I really do want to be like her and scream, "Where's Gary!"

But I don't want him to resent me or be embarrassed. Instead, I choose to wait for the spotlight. I walk up and down the aisle, wishing for the spotlight to shine. It does a couple of times but I don't see Gary. I still don't yell. My instincts tell me to try the other aisle of the auditorium. I stand midway down the aisle, in the pitch black, and wait. Within a second, the spotlight goes on again, with enough diffused light to illuminate Gary's face. He is right in front of me! Deep down I do not believe my standing in that exact location and the exact timing of the spotlight is a coincidence. I look up and murmur under my breath, "Thank you."

"Mom, what are you doing here?" he whispers, almost shouting.

"We've got to go." I tilt my head in the direction of the door and whisk him away.

On the drive to Hartford, Gary and Grandma marvel at the maple trees' leaves changing to shades of red. "You know, Gary," Grandma says as we pass an orange oak tree on the Merritt Parkway, "fall is my favorite season." I think she knows she is helping me by keeping Gary's mind off the doctor's visit.

But the truth is, taking Grandma anywhere adds an extra dimension to the outing. And taking her to Children's Hospital complicates things further. Besides adding in extra time for her to walk, I have to help her not break down from seeing all the sick children in the waiting areas. "When you were little, I used to thank God I was not sitting with you in a hospital. Now this! To see my little girl have to go through this!" She says this every couple of steps, just when she catches her breath. Even though she is huffing and puffing, her voice carries as if she is speaking into the hospital sound system. The other parents just stare at me. Gary is intentionally walking 10 steps ahead of us.

I roll my eyes, when she can't see my face, and say nothing to her. Does she think I did not pray enough and this is why I am here with my son? It's my fault? It's a conversation not worth having, because if I make that statement, she'll just break down and cry because I'm being so callous about her feelings. So I assume she doesn't mean it that way, instead of confronting her. When it comes to my mother, sometimes avoidance is the best medicine.

"She's crazy and it's hysterical, Mom," Gary chuckles as I scoot up to him to get away from her. I love that he loves her for who she is and that many times over the years he asks me "How'd you grow up with this?" He sees the difference between us. It's one of the many advantages of a multigenerational family. The kids gain a deeper appreciation for who you are and understand the life cycle more clearly. Besides, she leaves the occasional bed-pillow-chocolate as a way of showing her appreciation.

I leave Grandma in the waiting area as Gary and I are told to enter exam room number four. I turn around to reassure my mom.

"We'll be just a few minutes," I say. I see her crying on the chair at the sight of a painfully thin child.

The process for the doctor's appointment is consistent: Check in, and confirm insurance has not changed. Go with the nurse who weighs and measures the patient. Then, wait in the exam room. In the G.I. exam room, there is a huge color poster of the digestive system. Gary no longer kills time tracing his finger, as if it's a piece of food through a maze, reciting each organ, along the way. It's a game he's played far too many times. Eventually, the doctor enters the exam room.

Dr. Simmon's easy-going smile is missing. He talks directly to Gary.

"Hi. You've grown three quarters of an inch and gained three pounds," he says as a hello. Gary bursts with a smile. I sense the doctor is starting off with the positive but instead of letting Gary relish this growth, he launches directly into, "I've looked over your CT scan from yesterday and your Crohn's disease has progressed. Your current medication, Pentasa, will not be working for you anymore." He says it so quick without asking Gary any questions about his health or school or yesterday's E.R. visit.

My heart seems to stop. It's progressing? I thought he was managing it just fine. I didn't consider it would get worse. Crohn's is a digestive disorder that lasts a lifetime. There is no cure. Just more and more medications to keep it under control. If the medications stop working the doctors surgically remove more and more diseased intestines. Sometimes so much intestine is removed that patients live with a bag at their side for emptying their bowels. Sometimes the medications cause cancer. The doctor must have had a sense of the path my son's life would take but he's never discussed this with us. He handed us pamphlets initially. One was a cartoon book for Gary. I made calls to friends to try to understand the disease. It seemed everyone had a different story. The Internet just scared me with too much detail. I didn't know what to believe so I just did what the doctor ordered.

I am now in a little shock and try to listen carefully. Dr. Simmon starts rambling about two new medications, 6-MP and Remicade to relieve these new symptoms. What new symptoms? He explains both medications will help reduce inflammation and that Gary can eat anything he likes. There are side effects with the medications and he hands me a five-page stapled description of Remicade. As he tells Gary this is "one of the best medications," I glance down and see listed increased risk of cancer. My heart sinks. He says something about Gary losing his hair with 6-MP. Truth is, I barely hear anything except for this small remark: "With continued nutritional therapy, Gary will be limited with his foods."

I have no idea what Gary is thinking and when I look at him and he blurts out, "My friends are on Remicade. They are doing great, Mom." These are the friends he made at a six-day summer camp for kids called Camp Oasis funded by the Crohn's and Colitis Foundation of America. His camp friends keep in touch on Facebook. Now, they are influencing his choices. He just wants no pain and to fit in. I want to throw up. "Everybody has one" might be an argument a teenager makes for wanting a PlayStation. Parents know the response, "If they all jumped off the Brooklyn Bridge, would you?" But now, I have a doctor following protocol, a kid in pain and camp friends all pointing in one direction, the one I'll nickname the *cancer-causing cure*.

I actually gag. Dr. Simmon sees me hold my mouth and calmly says, "We have options for new medications and we don't have to decide today. In the meantime, Gary should take these two oral antibiotics. He should have an ultrasound downstairs and come back next Monday to see if the antibiotics are working. We don't have to decide this today. Just go downstairs, get an ultrasound and I'll see you next week." He rises to walk out the door and turns back, mentioning, "Oh, Gary, if you feel a puff of air when you urinate, call me immediately."

"OK, thanks," Gary says as Dr. Simmon rushes off to the next patient. He spent less than 15 minutes with us.

Gary puts on his sneakers and we stop by the waiting area for Grandma. Thankfully, she is no longer crying. She smiles at us. We explain that Gary needs to get an ultrasound. Somehow she knows not to ask if everything is all right in front of Gary. As he heads off in front of us again, she clutches her cane, slowly moving and whispering, "What he'd say?"

I try to be positive. If I break down, she'll fall apart. Then, I will have two patients.

"There are solutions to helping Gary so he is not in pain. There are medications. He gave me this paper to review." I hand it to her and she stops to put it in her almost worn-out oversized brown canvas bag. She likes feeling needed and giving her control of paperwork makes her feel good.

We head to the first floor for the ultrasound, slowly passing waiting rooms with sick children. The ultrasound waiting room is busy with moms pointing out the clownfish in the tank to their toddlers. "It's Nemo," exclaims one cute curly-brown-haired toddler with a bandage covering where something or other was put into or taken from her arm.

Gary checks in at the desk himself. "You stay with Grandma. I've done this before," he announces as he heads off for the scan.

As Gary is undergoing the ultrasound, my Mom and I sit in the waiting area surrounded by three little kids. My mom is welling up at the site of youngsters having to spend time in a hospital. Instead of saying anything at loudspeaker volume, she starts to read a page of the document about Remicade. She reads three-quarters of the first page and the tears drip down her cheek.

"I'll have to die before he takes this stuff. Your father would never allow it," she announces. It's almost like I am the teenager making this choice and she is using that same old tried and true mothering technique – guilt. I'm supposed to just give in to make my mother happy. Basically she is screaming at me. The other mothers turn their heads. I take the paper and read. The literature mentions cancer as a possible outcome. But the pros do seem convincing: Many Crohn's sufferers finally reach remission. Their pain and diarrhea diminish.

How am I going to get him to choose the right path? What is the right path? That sick feeling in my stomach returns. I always gave in to my mom's guilt technique. But, Gary is a different kid. He fights for what he thinks is right. I'm torn. I know I can't demand him to choose the nutritional therapy because if he doesn't want to do it, he'll sneak food and it will never work. But, no way am I going to let them pump him full of poison when he can try nutritional therapy first. According to Dr. Simmon, not everyone even has this option.

Gary tried nutritional therapy when he was first diagnosed to get the Crohn's in remission and to reduce the frequency of bowel movements. He knows it is tough, very tough. He did not eat for 30 days. He only drank a special supplement. As a middle-school student, imagine no birthday cake at a party; no pizza when the kids hang out. School lunchtime consisted of only a can of Ensure, while the other kids finished their chocolate chip cookies. Gary confided in me that the peer pressure was enormous. "C'mon you can have one small bite. Go ahead. Smell it." Kids can be cruel.

The first time Gary tried the therapy, I drew on a sheet of paper a table with 30 boxes and numbered them sequentially. During the day, he'd drink 10 cans of Ensure. At night he'd check off that he'd made it through the day. For incentive, I told him he could have a paint-ball party at the month's end, so in addition to checking off the box he'd write down the name of a friend he'd like to invite. By the end of the first week, he liked seeing his progress on the paper but he was tired all of the flavors, even his favorite, chocolate. By the last week, he'd stare at food circulars in the newspaper and drool at pictures of steak the same way other boys ogle at swimsuit models in Sports Illustrated. Now, at 15 he's headstrong and doesn't want me telling him what to do. Not even paintball parties are an incentive. He's old enough to make his own decisions. I sense at this point, in his mind it's Remicade.

Gary finishes the ultrasound. When he jumps into the car he says, "I don't know what I'm going to do. I have to think about it. Let's go." He doesn't have to urinate, he feels fine. He seems excited to go to the Chowder Pot. It's as if he doesn't have a care in the world. I think he just wants to forget everything and enjoy lunch. He's mastered the "shake it off" technique from his football days. Like my husband, Gary expresses little drama, a sharp contrast to my mom. Like many females, my mother likes discussing every-thing and wants to know *NOW* that Gary will not be taking the "*can-cer-causing cure.*" There is total silence in the car and I drive the short distance to the restaurant. My mom is rarely quiet, so I know she is trying to stay calm. But, just by looking at her fading color, I sense her heart is racing. It's a Venus and Mars situation and I feel the gravitational pull in both directions. I feel like I might break.

We sit down and look over the menus. Gary breaks the silence with, "I need to talk to my friends, Mom. You can't tell me what to do." I hadn't said a word.

Grandma, finally breaking her silence, uses her unique mother-ing techniques and pipes in, "Look, your mother would not have put her father through this. She would have just listened. There is no way Grandpa would want you on Remicade. How could you even consider other options?" For once, I don't mind her guilt technique. I figure maybe she could use it on him even though I hate it. I feel sick to my stomach – again – but I don't know what else to do. I stay quiet.

The lobster arrives and Gary puts on the plastic bib as if nothing is wrong. Based on all our other visits, I know all he wants to do is pull off the claws and look to see how much meat is in this one. He wants to separate the head and look for the red roe, to make sure it is a female. (They're sweeter.) He wants to take off the legs, place them on the plate and take the big piece of meat out of the tail. He wants to cut each piece in equal size pieces, then dunk them one at a time in the melted butter and eat. His precision is a telling aspect of his personality.

"Can't we just enjoy lunch already?" he pleads with us. But neither my Mom nor I have mastered the "shake it off" technique. We try. Uncharacteristically, we quietly eat lunch. We quietly drive home. We quietly suffer with the realization of the disease progression. Gary quietly goes up to his room to start his homework.

I go downstairs to my office and call an acquaintance, Ruth Hill, a 50-something pleasant woman who smiles easily. Her husband died from complications of Crohn's disease. Ruth has a photography business in town and we are a part of the same business networking group. Over the years, we've shared stories about elder care and child care but never really discussed Crohn's or the death of her husband.

"Ruth, I know this is personal and you may not want to share details with me," I start, not knowing how to continue. I blurt out, "Gary's Crohn's disease is progressing and I need to help him get information to make a choice."

"Oh, Randi, I'm so sorry. I didn't realize he has Crohn's," she says. There is a genuine warmth to her tone.

"I know I've mentioned it … I understand if you don't want to share your experience," I say, trying to emulate her warmth. She jumps right in.

"Randi, let me tell you. My husband was diagnosed at age 17. Back then they put him on prednisone. It's a steroid. Those things are vicious. Watch out for them. I don't think they use them today," she says. I think to myself I wish that were the case, but we're still using the same things. She continues, "The standard line you hear is we have to deal with today."

"I've heard that said."

"Through the years it was one complication after another. But we dealt with 'today.' The best time he had was for a couple of years when he watched his diet. He lost weight and felt great. But eventually the Crohn's came back and he ended up on painkillers and other medications," she says. "When he got cancer I asked the doctor to please take him off the medications, because his personality was so erratic. He was hard to live with. I didn't recognize his personality anymore. And the doctor said, 'We have to deal with what we have today. Do you want me to deal with his pain or the cancer?' Randi, he died six months later."

I don't remember the rest of the conversation. I cry. I tell her I'm sorry. I hang up the phone and go up to Gary's room. He is doing his bio homework.

"What's up, Mom?" He sounds like he's been focused on school work. I need to break my silence with him and share what I've learned.

"You mentioned that you wanted to get input from other people to help with your decision? I just spoke to Ruth. She's willing to talk to you."

"What she'd say?" he asks.

"Are you sure you want me to tell you?"

"Yeah."

I relate the story to him and he cries, the first tears I've seen since he was diagnosed three years earlier. I hug him, like when he was a little boy, and he doesn't flinch away. I wipe my tears off his cheek.

"I don't know what I am going to do, Mom. I'd give anything to have a normal body."

"I know, Gary. I don't know why this happened to you. But you have options. You can try one approach and if it doesn't work you can always try another."

"Mom, I'm going to hang out in my room tonight," he says. My heart breaks for him.

"I love you, Gary. I'll see you in the morning."

"I love you too."

Unlike last night, I doubt either of us will sleep well.

What You Can Do Now

---

1. Make a game out of a procedure.

Don't tell your loved one they have to do something. Find a way to make it fun. I like making boxes and checking off progress. So, whether you can't eat for 30 days or have to drink barium in 30 minutes, breaking it down into small pieces and seeing the accomplishment by X-ing out the milestone builds momentum. Build up your loved one's confidence. Do not tear them down. Let them decide how to break up the goal into manageable pieces. By giving them a voice, they will have more ownership to accomplish the goal. Build in a reward at the end.

2. Stay calm.

Have trust that the simple things will take care of themselves. When I needed to find Gary in the dark auditorium, I choose not to create a ruckus. By staying calm, I found him. I also took a second to acknowledge how grateful I was for the spotlight.

3. Get your options in writing.

If you're getting worse, ask the doctor for information on your options. After he or she informs you, ask if there are any others. Get a complete list. This is how I discovered a nutritional option for Gary. I found I couldn't retain what was said to me in the exam room, but having information sheets helped me understand the options better. If the doctor does not have materials on hand, write down the correct spelling of the options and search on the Internet. If it is not an emergency and a decision is not needed imminently, learn as much as you can before you commit to a course of action.

* * *

Chapter 4
Pee Pain, Pillows and Processes

I hear the floor creak outside my bedroom door. The sound is so faint, even Chloe the dog doesn't stir. But I am wide awake. I listen harder and the door knob turns. I look at the clock. It reads 2:24 a.m. In the pitch black, I barely can make out Gary's outline. He sneaks next to my bedside and seems scared.

"Mom, I just peed and I felt a puff of air. It hurt like hell." He whispers this. I think he doesn't want to wake his dad.

"OK, I'll call the doctor," I say as I jump up out of bed. My only direction from the doctor, earlier in the day, was if there was a puff of air when Gary peed, to call the hospital. Steve stirs in bed and I tell him I'm going downstairs for the phone number to call the doctor.

In the dark, I miss the first step, and yell out in fright, while simultaneously grabbing onto the railing to prevent me rolling downstairs. Grandma, who can't seem to remember anything but hears everything, and never sleeps at night, detects the commotion on the stairs and screams, "What's going on?"

Now, even Chloe is barking. Steve races to me on the stairs and as I look up I see Matt dashing to Grandma's side to comfort her.

I pull myself up and race downstairs for our phone book and place the call. The phone number rings through, first time, and the doctor's answering service doesn't even have me wait for the on-call doctor to return the call. They patch me through immediately. When the doctor takes the call, all I say is "puff of air" and she orders me to bring Gary to the emergency room in Hartford, now, so he can to be seen by the G.I. doctors.

When I call the doctor and they tell me to go to the emergency room, I assume it is an emergency. So I tell her, "The Children's Hospital in Hartford is an hour-and-a-half trip from our house! Maybe we should go closer?"

"No. Drive carefully but come, here, now," she says. "He needs to be at Children's Hospital."

The word "now" echoes in my mind. Dr. Simmon did not say why it was a big deal to pee air, so I feel clueless. I instruct my husband to pack an overnight bag for Gary and for me. While he is racing between rooms, filling the bag with toothbrushes, change of underwear and clothes, I stand alone, in my bedroom closet, feeling dread. I take three deep breaths. I put on my most comfortable sweat pants and lace up my most comfortable sneakers. I grab my well-worn fall coat from the closet, pick off some of the horse hay, and watch it fall to the floor. I see Matt, who I'm afraid is basically raising himself as I try to help Gary with this disease. I put on my super calm voice and tell him softly to go back to his room and to go to sleep. "I'll call you before you leave for school in the morning," I say, and give him a quick kiss.

I walk downstairs and Steve hands me the overstuffed overnight bag. He stands next to the door and I look directly in his eyes. He needs no words to tell me his thoughts. I see his love. We just stare at each other for a brief second. As I hold the canvas bag, he wraps his big arms around me and holds me close, and squeezes me a little too tight. I drop the bag and hug him back. Then he turns to Gary and gives him a kiss on the forehead. Gary and I race to the garage. After I turn on the car ignition, I realize I forgot to say goodbye to Grandma. I am too panicked to be concerned about her.

It is 2:50 a.m. when I pull out of the driveway and use my high beams to watch out for the night critters. There are no overhead lights on our street, and a moonless night is especially dark. I spy a skunk casually crossing the road and I slam on the brakes. To get there fast, I'm going to have to drive slow.

"Mom, we've never been outside at this time of night. Be careful," Gary warns. His voice is calm, almost like he doesn't want to make me more nervous.

We head onto the Merritt Parkway, which during rush hour I call the "Park it" Parkway from all the congestion. It's as if daylight comes instantly on the parkway, but without the traffic. Intense lights illuminate the road for highway crews to work all night. I squint to stay in the lane with bright yellow cones on one side and concrete dividers on the other. With construction, the lanes are narrower than usual. I want to race up to the hospital, but can't because the lane is too tight, the police seem to be everywhere and the workers tend to stand right next to the edge of the yellow cones. I feel like I am crawling in traffic even though no one else is on the road. I turn on a Jim Brickman CD. He's a piano soloist who plays meditative melodies that calm my nerves. Gary tries to make light conversation. "Can you believe how few people are on the road, Mom?"

"How about we count how many cars until Hartford?" I say as if we are on an adventure. He isn't in pain; he went to the bathroom before we left. We just need to deal with the puff of air. I know I should help him stay In The Moment to keep us calm.

I figure counting cars is a good diversion, but before we start counting I ask him, "Know why I am not nervous driving right now?" I try to make a teachable moment, hoping something good can come from this. Most of the time, my kids hate my stories. They have either heard them before or the point seems too obvious. They roll their eyes so I can see their "here she goes again" thoughts. They see me roll my eyes at my Mom too, but I at least do it behind her back! I wait for Gary's response to see if he's engaged.

"Nope."

Ahh, the monosyllabic speak again. I sort of hate it but it's typical and, considering the circumstances, I am grateful he is not hysterical. That would make driving unbearable.

"Did I ever tell you about the time dad had back surgery and I drove home to feed our old dog, Misty?" I already knew I never shared this story with him; I've been keeping it for the appropriate time, like now. I figure, at least he won't roll his eyes thinking "not this one again."

"Nope."

I continue.

"Well, about a year after our car accident – when Dad and I were hit by a drunk driver, before you were born – Dad needed surgery on his slipped disk because his pain was so bad. The doctors squeezed in his surgery on New Year's Eve. The procedure took much longer than expected. I stayed with him in recovery. Foolishly, I hadn't made arrangements for Misty so I had to go home to walk her. Remember Misty?"

"Yep," he says. He is still with me and I think he, too, likes talking about something else.

"So I had to drive home. It was 10 o'clock at night, in a snow storm. The roads were slippery, the plows hadn't come yet and I swerved all over the place. The windshield wipers barely kept up with the snow," I say, making it sound as terrifying as it felt to me.

"Were you scared?" he says. At least he's asking questions.

"Yes, Gary. I was nervous about the road conditions, worried that my husband might have trouble walking and couldn't understand why I needed to be on the freeway on a night with drunk drivers. Especially after I was hit by a drunk driver and was almost killed. It seemed too much for me. I asked God why I had such a challenge and got no answer… Until now."

I pause.

"Huh?" Gary says.

"You see, right now I am driving my son at 3:00 a.m." I point to the digital clock on the dashboard and I see him gaze down, like the precise time is etched in our lives together forever, and continue, "I have no idea what is really wrong with you. But, I am grateful it is not snowing. It could be worse. If I hadn't gone through the other experience, I think this would be overwhelming for me. Now, I know I have the inner strength to drive carefully with so much on my mind. I've done it before and I can do it again. I know it could be worse."

We drive in silence, except for the occasional sound of a jack-hammer on the side of the road. Gary breaks the silence. "Mom, so why do you think I have to go through this?"

Ah, the question I ask every day.

"I don't know. But I know that as nervous as you are now, the doctors will help you and you will be fine. My guess is the next time you see 3:00 a.m. on a car clock you will remember this moment. You'll find strength from this experience and be a stronger man for it." I think this sounds credible because I really believe it.

Gary says, "This isn't so bad. It could be worse. I could have to pee and it could be snowing." Without ever rolling his eyes, Gary closes them and sleeps the rest of the car ride.

I pull into the emergency room around 4 a.m. Gary and I walk up to the admitting attendant, a 30-ish woman who looks tired, bloated and like she wishes she were home asleep. Because Gary does not have to pee, he is not in pain. He is not flushed nor does he look like he has any symptoms of the dreaded flu. We are so calm, she looks at us perplexed, and wonders why we are here bothering her.

"The doctor told us to come. Immediately," I say, like the red carpet should be waiting for us. It's an emergency, right?

She checks to see if there was a call from a doctor and if our name is in the system. "No mention of a call." She says this like we are "D" list players and she enjoys her superiority. Without information in the system she looks at us like we are wasting her time.

"Please call the doctor to let her know we are here," I say, forcing myself to use the calm voice. I'm thinking, after all, it's an emergency. That's why we were told to leave immediately and not wait for the sun to rise. Is my kid's bladder going to burst? Is the pee poisoning his body? Is there a tear in something somewhere? I have no idea.

The attendant calls the on-call doctor and from our end of the conversation it sounds like she wakes the doctor up from a sound sleep. After a brief exchange the attendant hands me the phone and the doctor says, groggily, "Great, I am glad you made it. They will take care of you." She hangs up the phone and I realize I don't even know her name.

A triage nurse takes Gary and me to her station. We are all familiar with this process: health insurance first and then patient symptoms. With a couple of keystrokes she finds Gary's record in the system. We confirm our insurance carrier, address and Gary's allergies. In response to the question of why are we here, Gary describes his pain when he urinates, in a precise, factual way. "It's a 12 on a 1 to 10 scale and takes 20 minutes for the pain to subside." He eliminates any drama with his description and tells her he has not gone fully in at least six hours. The nurse nods like she understands and mentions "a catheter can eliminate fluids for you." Seeing his quizzical look, she continues, "The catheter is inserted into your penis so you can urinate."

"I don't want that," Gary says, "I'll tell you that right now. Does it hurt?" With three statements in a row, I know he is nervous.

The nurse is wearing a Looney Toons cartoon-emblazoned medical uniform. She has a soft voice but it is deep, like she can get control of any situation. My guess is she has years of experience with screaming kids. I think she also knows the picture of Daffy Duck doesn't fool anybody.

Her voice turns firm. "You want it straight?"

"Yep." I detect a little quiver in his voice.

"It hurts like heck. I've never met anyone who likes getting a catheter." She uses the deepest part of her range to share this information.

Gary crosses his legs. I know it hurts like hell for him to pee. Not understanding the air factor makes it even scarier, never mind a catheter.

"You'll have to wait to be seen," she says. "Please go to the waiting room."

The waiting room is brightly lit, with "The Lion King" blaring on the TV to an audience of no one. So much for the swine flu epidemic. The night guard is laughing with the night cleaning man, who is washing the floors with a very noisy machine. You'd never know it's the middle of the night.

"How long do you think we'll be waiting?" Gary asks me. I think because he sees no one he expects to be seen immediately. But my experience tells me differently.

"At least one hour, I bet. Notice there are no clocks here? Look around. See any?" I watch him turn around 360 degrees searching every wall for a clock. He sees lots of brightly colored animal paintings, but he shakes his head indicating no clocks anywhere.

"Know why?"

"Nope."

"Time is irrelevant at this point. If you focus on how long things take you'll get frustrated. These are professionals; they know when time is really urgent. So, we have all the time now." I lie down on a couch and he goes to the other couch. My handbag is an uncomfortable pillow and my coat shields the blaring florescent light from my tired eyes but "Hakuna Matata" blares an unwelcome lullaby.

After about five minutes, I hear Gary get up. I peek out from under my coat and watch him walk to the restroom. I cover my head back up with the coat. About 10 minutes pass and he is not back. I start to get nervous. I don't hear him yelling, because the floor waxing machine is going full blast, the Lion King is roaring and the bathroom is far from where I am trying to rest. I am just about to get up to go knock on the door when I see him walking toward me, looking relieved.

"Mom, I emptied my bladder. It hurt like hell. It's empty, though. They don't have to put in a catheter. I did see blood but I don't care – no catheter." He looks relieved but in pain. He goes to the couch and covers his head with his sweatshirt. I cover my head again with my coat. Blood? If I felt anything it would be numb.

Two hours later we're summoned. A baby screams and screams in the room next to ours. It is relentless. Gary cringes at hearing the pain of the baby and I feel bad for the mom. But as much as I understand her pain, I have to focus on my son. No one comes in to take Gary's vitals or anything. We just wait, trying to shut our eyes and get some rest. Finally, a woman comes in to the room and asks if we want pillows and a blanket. Just looking at her outfit, I don't think she is a nurse. She looks like someone responsible for taking out the trash, but she seems to understand we are in a crisis and a little attention would help. I want to hug her.

She appears a couple of minutes later and, like magic, hands over some pillows and a blanket. I prop the pillows on the chair and cover myself with the blanket. Gary sees me a little more comfortable on my makeshift bed of two chairs and smiles at me. He closes his eyes. It feels like seconds later, someone turns on the lights. She says she is a nurse and hooks Gary up to an I.V. for antibiotics. I am too tired to question her. She seems to be fresh, like she just started the shift, and is cheerful. With the same excitement as "You've just won a free cruise!" she says, "You'll be admitted to the hospital!"

Even Gary knows not to ask when.

Gary's never been admitted before and I feel like I am hiking in the woods without a path. I've lost track of time and am confused by the goings on. There seem to be so many new faces, all with specific jobs. I can't figure out one person's role from another. I feel tired, confused. Frantic. Not the best combination to think clearly for my son.

To help me put this all in context, I search for a business analogy. Maybe this will calm me. What business is this similar too? I think about the positions I've held in GE. This doesn't seem to be anything like manufacturing new aircraft instruments. In that business, I spent endless hours in meetings with the customer – the engine manufacturers – discussing every aspect of the design and its impact on an engine. My team lived in fear knowing that any change we made would affect engine performance and, if done incorrectly, could cause a crash.

I think about my time as the program manager for the design phase of the electronic combat system for the Stealth Fighter. Even though I held a top secret military clearance, communication on the team was fluid, only it happened behind closed steel doors in a windowless room. I made sure everyone knew every process and step we needed to make. I even challenged both the generals of the Navy and Air Force to agree on requirements so we could meet their needs and complete the job on time and budget. At that time, they were not used to answering to a woman, but they did it. It was clear; I was the point of contact for the program.

But not here in the hospital. I can't figure out who is in charge. And it sure isn't me.

My thoughts are interrupted when an attendant comes with a wheelchair for Gary. Watching him, I realize the attendant is like the bell hop at a hotel. Instead of taking your bags, he transports patients and the I.V. He provides door-to-door transport, wiggling the I.V. cords around the wheelchair and into the elevator, instead of finagling too many bags. Finding comfort with the hotel analogy, I continue gaining context. The concierge is the nurse ready to help you 24/7. The décor is brightly colored cartoon animals on walls, instead of wide windows for gazing upon views of a golf course and pool. Both places change sheets and have room service. Both places want you to feel good. With this context, and my business acumen, I make myself feel a little more comfortable in my new surroundings.

As the attendant pushes the sixth-floor elevator button, I'm actually just as excited as when waiting for a hotel room in the lobby for hours and they finally announce, "Your room is ready." Gary, too, looks excited to be going up to his room. Now, Gary will see his doctor, he will receive care, he'll have his own room to rest and he'll get better.

The overzealous hellos from the nurses on the floor remind me of the enthusiasm hotel staff show at the check-in desk. The attendant swings open the oversized wooden door to Gary's room. I quickly glance in and see a hospital bed with steel bars on both sides and monitoring equipment. It is stark, clean and impersonal. I feel I've entered the twilight zone because I realize I am not in control of when we get to check out.

Gary focuses right in on the flat screen TV and DVD player and announces, "Look at the latest technology!" He turns his head to see the rest of the room and shouts, "I've got my own bathroom, Mom! This is better than home!" He's showing his true Oster characteristics of making lemonade from lemons.

I force out a "Great!" I try not to sound cynical but I don't think I hit upbeat either. I'm exhausted.

It's pretty much of a whirlwind for the next couple of hours. Lots of people enter the room, some touching Gary, some cleaning the sink, some looking at monitors. It's noisy in here. Gary is hooked up to several machines. Neither one of us knows what they do. Gary still hasn't been seen by a doctor. No one explains anything. On top of the new sounds and smells is the continuous ring of my cellphone. The calls are from family and friends, basically wondering the same thing: "Everything all right? What's going on? How long will he be there? How's he feeling? Did the doctor say anything? What is the prognosis?" I wish I knew the answer to any or all of these questions but I don't. My job is to try to keep everyone calm.

My husband needs to work and feels guilty for not being here. He has to go to New Jersey for a few days. They fired the administrator for the New Jersey surgical center and Steve has taken over the job as of today. They're calling it a promotion, to go from managing one surgical center to two, 150 miles apart from each other.

But they are only giving him 5 percent more in pay. So, it's more like work expansion. It beats the alternative, a layoff. It is sad for me to admit this but we need his family health insurance coverage right now more than we need him to be here in the hospital room.

My mom calls too. "You know," she says, "Steve's side of the family gave him this disease." I just roll my eyes. I don't know where she gets these things. This is one of those times I wish I had a sibling, so we could commiserate. Gary turns down the volume of the TV and interrupts me on another call. "Mom," he says, "I have to pee. Don't be mad if you hear me cursing. It's how I get through the pain."

"No problem, Gary. Do what you have to do," I say while answering the same questions with Gary's uncle, Jay.

A nurse, relatively young and with a pleasant demeanor, is in the room. She must think I'm a callous bitch because I am not fawning over Gary. But I know I'm not helping him any by falling apart every time he pees. The nurse turns off one of the beeping machines and asks Gary what his current pain level is.

"It's a five on a scale of 1 to 10. It never seems to go below that but escalates real fast during and after peeing." He seems to like the factual way the nurses record pain. It's not dramatic.

"Would you say it gets to 10?" she politely asks.

"12. You'll see," he says, actually sounding eager to show her what he's been going through. She unplugs him from the two machines and he rolls another one with him into his bathroom. I stare at him until he shuts the bathroom door. I can't believe he is not complaining or feeling sorry for himself. Instead he just gets to his business.

"FUCK. OH FUCK," he screams. It seems that with each rising point on the pain scale Gary's volume rises until he is yelling so loud, my stomach sinks. I'm shaking to each "Fuck." It is like a double-edged knife stabbing my heart. I hate seeing Gary suffer. No child should have to go through this. I want to burst through the door and inhabit his body so I can absorb the pain for him. The young nurse, who to me seems minutes out of high school, looks at me and tries to comfort me with "He'll be OK." Somehow in my exhausted state I don't start ranting, "How do you know? Where the hell is the doctor? How long will Gary be here?" Instead, I just try to appear confident. "I hope so," I say.

I'm not sure how long I'll be able to keep it together. I lost it once before on one of his ambulance rides. I was sitting in the passenger's seat. I poked my head in the back of the ambulance when Gary finally came to. Gary pointed to me and asked the EMT, "Who is this?" He did not recognize me, not a clue who I was. The young ambulance driver, sitting next to me, covered in tattoos, said in a matter-of-fact voice that this was typical seizure reaction. The ambulance driver was reciting seizure symptoms with the same emotion as if he were saying when you have a cold, your nose runs. Only he left out, "lady," with an eye roll, at the end of the sentence. I felt like I'd just lost my child. How could Gary not know who I was? He looked at me like I was a stranger. At that point to Gary, there was no difference between the EMT and me in terms of our relationship. Actually, he probably thought the EMT could help him better than I could. I was a bystander. I couldn't lash out at the EMT because he had more skills than I had to help Gary. So I broke down and sobbed, out-of-control crying where I couldn't even stand up. When Gary didn't recognize me, it was the worst feeling of my life. Now, hearing him scream and moan is a close second.

Gary finishes his business and rolls his apparatus out of the bathroom. Once he stops urinating the pain subsides significantly, but doesn't disappear. But it does dissipate enough that he can take a standing ovation from the nurse. I think he thinks she's cute.

"So, I can tell you hit a level 12 for pain. How are you now?" she says as she starts to hook back up his pumping machines.

"An eight. It will start to go down. I think I am going to rest." As he climbs back into the bed, he turns to me and continues, "Mom, can you drive home and get my backpack? I have homework to do and a bio lab report."

I know if I say don't worry about the report, he'll feel as if I've given up on him. He wants to keep his life as normal as possible. I remember at one Crohn's conference a psychologist told the parents that our children will live in pain. If we comfort them every time they complain, they will learn to use it as an excuse. They will become weak. He used the butterfly analogy with the chrysalis, the story where the little boy helps the butterfly break out of the chrysalis by opening it for the insect. The butterfly dies afterward because the butterfly needed to struggle to gain strength to survive in the world. The doctor explains that these kids need to learn to achieve in spite of the pain. His message was very clear: "Don't baby them."

Well I must have gotten an "F" in that lecture because now I want to say to Gary, "Are you nuts? You are in the hospital. The teacher will understand. You were just screaming in pain." But instead I follow Gary's lead and I decide to drive home to pick up the backpack. We haven't seen a doctor all day, and no one seems to know when the doctor will be stopping by to see Gary. According to the nurse, it might not be until tonight. I figure I will take Grandma and Matthew back to the hospital with me. This way they can visit Gary and we can eat dinner at the hospital. Grandma likes to eat dinner every night at 6 p.m. There is no way I can cook dinner for them tonight. If the timing works, I'll have them in the hospital cafeteria around six. I need to get things as regular as possible to keep my mom calm – which enables me to focus on Gary. Matt will have to give my mom her eye drops. I am trying my best to support everybody and feel like I am doing nothing well, since I realize I forgot to call Matt this morning before school started.

I pick up my purse to leave for the 90-minute drive home for Gary's backpack. Just as I am walking out the door, a different nurse enters the room. I know she is a nurse because she points up to a white bulletin board, permanently marked with the room and phone number. She writes in erasable green marker "Oct. 21" and next to "Nurse" she writes her name, "Casey." Behind her is a matronly 40-ish curly-haired blonde in a dark floral dress and comfortable shoes. Looking at the next item on the board, I ask, "Is she the P.C.A.? What is a P.C.A.?" I probably sound cranky.

The nurse doesn't say what a P.C.A. is but responds immediately. "Oh – no, she is Dr. Stark." Perhaps this is the doctor who told us to come to the emergency room in the middle of the night, but I am not sure. I am in overdrive at this point. But I know I've never seen her or heard her name before.

"Hi, I'm Dr. Stark. How are you?" I'm about to answer but she continues without skipping a beat. "I work with Dr. Simmon." She says this to me as she walks toward Gary. She continues, "Let me see how you are doing." She pushes down on Gary's belly the same way Gary's pediatrician and the other E.R. doctor touched him. He yelps "Ow!" the same way again. She takes out her stethoscope and listens to his heart. The "examination" takes less than three minutes.

She pulls up a chair next to the hospital bed and I sit on the couch. She explains that the I.V. antibiotics should kill off the infection. She says she likes to "cool off" the system before any next steps are taken. I have no idea what any of this means. I want to ask her but she keeps talking. It could take a couple of days and each day he should be in less pain. In about three minutes she seems to have determined a path for him. She smiles like she's on stage. The twilight zone sensation returns to me.

I am not sure where Gary's doctor is but clearly she is communicating with him. I find it unsettling not to see Dr. Simmon and not to understand even where he is in this picture. I sense Dr. Stark is very busy and she too will be flittering in and out. I have no idea what her background is and she doesn't offer any credentials other than that she's a doctor. I am supposed to just trust her. Wouldn't it be great if they had a bio sheet preprinted for each person entering the room? Even when you go to a play they tell you, with pride, who the performers are. But here, the people suddenly entering my life are mystery people. They rush in and out. I am stuck with my first impressions and no facts. Yet they are making critical life choices on behalf of my loved ones.

Dr. Stark continues. After the system "cools off," Gary will be *"an excellent candidate for surgery."*

What? Since when were we talking about surgery? And to accomplish what? Is this for the pee pain? Is it for Crohn's disease? Dr. Simmon never mentioned surgery, at least not at this juncture. I know that some people end up losing so much of their intestine they need a bag at their side for defecating. Is this the surgery she is referring to? Is Gary's condition worse than they ever told me? I stare at her. I feel so lost. I don't understand the disease, the terminology, the progression. I know I am not stupid, but I certainly feel dumb now. I can't even figure out what questions to ask. I take a deep breath. I walk to the sink for a cup of water to gain time. I've learned that during a crisis is not the best time to make informed decisions. It is even harder to think rationally with my child screaming in pain. I will do anything anyone says to get him better. I've prayed to give me the pain instead. It's killing me watching him suffer.

My child is certainly not the first to need surgery. Still, I feel like I am melting under pressure. Where is my release valve? Why does this feel so sudden? In GE we worked so hard to identify problems early in a process so that we avoided worst-case scenarios. The mantra was NO SURPRISES. This way, we were always prepared for the possibility of bad news. In my engineering days, if the aircraft was flying in the desert, we planned for outrageous heat. Even after we figured out the safety factor to cope with heat, we'd double the factor just to make sure we were covered. Doubling wasn't a scientific methodology, just basic engineering to ensure we planned for worst case and then unexpected case. How does a person get to this point in parenting, without ever realizing surgery is an option for their child?

Where is the play-book for patients and families? What is the process? Where are the case histories of others with the disease and outcomes? I've heard over and over from doctors that every case is different. I get that each person is unique, I even like this concept. But, my Bronx roots are not buying it. Gary cannot be so different from other Crohn's patients that there was no way to tell surgery would be needed. My skepticism is supported by my statistics background that recalls the theory of a normal distribution curve. Yes, there are outsiders, but most people fall into the "norm." What is the "norm" for Crohn's? How can I make decisions without facts? And why is a new option thrown in at the last minute by a person I just met?

In order to evaluate options, I need to know the risks, benefits and long-term consequences. I have to compare options. This is not something that can be accomplished in a 15-minute meeting with a doctor. I need to learn. Someone has to talk to me, in depth. I need an expert's time. Where is my son's doctor? Where is anyone who can explain to me what Crohn's is? I am willing to learn and I understand the doctor's time is valuable, but this seems like a crisis – at least it is to my family.

Yet, this machine seems to keep on ticking without emotion and drama. Only my heart seems to be pounding outside my sweater. If I were slightly prepared, maybe I would feel more in control. And calmer. I would feel prepared for her quick, casual statement: *"an excellent candidate for surgery"*.

My hand shakes. I gulp the water. I feel the coldness travel down my esophagus. The reality is I need to be Gary's long-term advocate. A crisis doesn't really help me, help him. Somehow, I need to gain control. Dr. Stark looks at the machines and touches one of the bags. As she does her work, I recall how I went through this with my father during his final illness at age 79. He too was "an excellent candidate for surgery." I brought my dad to the emergency room because to me it looked like he'd had a stroke. He could not hold up his Carvel ice cream cup and his mouth was drooling and sagging. After 11 hours of waiting in the E.R. and undergoing a CT scan an attendant brought him up to a room. When the doctor entered the room my dad looked up, tilted his head, and quipped, "What's up, Doc?" I'll never forget it.

I was struck by my dad's calmness and his choice to sound like Bugs Bunny. The diagnosis was a brain tumor called a glioblastoma. Turns out this wasn't the kind of tumor that's round and solid and easily removed. It was more like tree roots growing throughout the brain. All I wanted was for my father to be fine. He was not sickly before this. He and my mom lived with us and took care of the kids while my husband and I worked more than full time. I was the major breadwinner of the family and felt the pressure of the "sandwich generation." My parents and my kids were the bread squishing me between work obligations. My job did not take a break for a personal crisis. I tried to balance corporate demands, children's demands and elder care, while keeping my husband happy. Sometimes, my life felt like a house of cards ready to implode. I feared a feather could take it down.

With my father sitting in his hospital bed, he told me he just wanted the facts about his prognosis and asked me to help him get them. My mom just held his hand and tried to hide her tears, as I stared at them both in a daze. My cellphone rang and brought me back to my work reality. It was my manager. She could tell I was not myself or at my desk working from home, like I said I was. I told her I was in the hospital with my dad. She, too, had been through medical emergencies and in unemotional corporate speak, she told me the best advice ever: "Randi, the doctors will only answer the questions you ask," she said. "They will not give you more information than you request. Don't be afraid to ask the hard questions." Before she hung up she told me to take care of my dad and that she'd handle the work stuff. I felt so appreciative of her support. Now, I just had my family to manage, at least for a day.

As I hung up the phone, a young female resident surgeon, perfectly thin, beautiful smile and oozing confidence, was meeting with my father telling him the doctor told her to tell him they scheduled brain surgery for the next day. I figured this must be the resident brain surgeon from Yale who the nurse had earlier mentioned. I figured the actual brain surgeon was equally impressive. I was impressed with the resident's quick implementation of the doctor's solution. The caliber of her education meant to me that she knew surgery was the best next step; otherwise wouldn't we be discussing other options? I automatically figured my dad was going to get the best care, which to me he deserved. He was a WWII vet, and lived a clean, hard-working, honest life. He deserved his dignity as he faced what could be his final illness. The resident quickly told me the brain surgeon would be stopping by later in the day to meet with my dad. I was thrilled. They would help him.

All day my dad kept saying he wanted a "minimally invasive approach" and did not want chemo and radiation. He kept saying this to anyone who'd listen but no one seemed to actually be listening, not even me. He was going down a path he said he didn't want, or at least didn't fully understand, but couldn't figure out how to slow the process. Lying in bed, he looked up at me almost as his last resort and asked again, "Can you please find out what the surgery entails?"

My parents, who just yesterday seemed perfectly fine, were in the middle of a medical crisis. Nothing really prepared me for it. I was their "little girl." Our roles reversed in that instant. Still in shock about the quick turn of my dad's health, I held back my tears and forced a smile. "Sure," I said.

By the time the brain surgeon showed up, hours later, my mom had worried herself into a state where she couldn't stand up without breaking down. I kept giving her tissues, some I'd used myself. My dad asked me to talk to the doctor without my mom present. My dad loved my mom's New York, pushy, mouthy, dramatic way, but knew it probably would not work in Connecticut, more of a string-pearl and soft voice state that emphasizes etiquette. Besides, at this point, she couldn't concentrate or retain any information and seemed to need more emotional support than my dad did.

I grabbed another tissue and stepped out into the hall with the doctor. I shut my dad's hospital room door and braced myself against the wall for support. I was pretending to be strong for the private discussion with the brain surgeon. The doctor's imposing frame next to my petite build was not ideal for level conversation, something I learned in GE was critical during negotiations. Many times I lost authority by being petite; I always looked for chairs to sit in to level the height disparity. But there were none in the narrow hall. The doctor had no choice but to look down on me. Instead of gaining control by acting calmly, showing the poise of a Fairfield County executive and introducing myself to the doctor, as I was trained to do in GE, I skipped that step. Instead, my own pushy New York ways combined with my boss' suggestion to ask the hard questions made me just blurt out, "How long will he live without surgery and how long with surgery?" I could not believe I was asking such a cold question. I felt a lump in my throat, and touched the wall with both hands behind my back.

The doctor smiled, as if he was proud he knew the answer, and said, "Simple: eight weeks without surgery and eight months with surgery." He continued with the fine-print speech. "There is a very good chance with brain surgery he could experience some paralysis on one side of his body. He might have trouble speaking. He probably won't see colors. Also, he'd still need chemo and radiation. He'd be home with the family so you could provide care at home, take him for treatments, and help him with pain from surgery."

That is exactly what my dad wanted to avoid. He didn't want to go back and forth for chemo. He knew from his testicular cancer, eight years earlier, that chemo was no picnic. Why would they schedule this surgery without asking him or heeding his wishes, I wondered.

Asking the hard question first provided me with the critical information: eight weeks versus eight months. "So," I said, "without surgery he could go home, have no additional pain, meet with his friends and family and slowly deteriorate. He will eventually fall asleep and not wake up. With surgery, he could be a vegetable, but maybe not. But he definitely will have pain, chemo, radiation and need after care, starting tomorrow?"

"Yes, but don't forget he'll also have time for *one last cruise*," the doctor said, sounding like a salesman to me. One last cruise reverberated in my head. My father should go through all of this pain for one last cruise? He'd lived 79 relatively healthy years and prided himself in knowing that he provided for his family, not the other way around. In the couple of minutes the doctor spent with my dad, he clearly did not know him. After the Navy, my dad never wanted to go on a ship again.

My dad elected not to have surgery and the hospital threw him out the next day. "There is nothing we can do for him," somebody said as they showed us the door. I am pretty sure the person was a social worker, one who made me feel like I did not love my dad because I was not doing *everything* to extend his life.

As I was leaving the next day, a resident pulled me aside in the hall. "I got to know your dad last night," he said. "He's a remarkable man and brave to make the choice he did." He hesitated and whispered, "You know, the doctors get $15,000 for the surgery and then it's $3,000 a day for after care. They don't tell you that."

We took my dad home. At the beginning, he was fully mobile. I invited his friends and relatives to the house and we spent the weekends laughing over old photo albums and memories. We celebrated his life. He had time and brain capacity to impart all his life wisdom to me. As the stairs became harder to navigate, my husband and I moved my dad's bed to my husband's first floor den, with its own bathroom. My boss even let me work from home. At the time, I was responsible for a new GE initiative to educate consumers on long-term care. GE was leading the first national long-term care awareness day and I frantically was negotiating with partners for Internet content and participation in the national event, an irony because as I worked, I cared for my dad. I'd take my conference calls in the den and be comforted by my dad's snoring. As he slept, I negotiated terms and conditions with other businesses. If he woke up and needed me, I'd be right there. My father could see my stress level because for the first time, he watched me work. One day, when I was juggling e-mails, conference calls, deadlines and my cellphone, he told me to stop.

"Come here," he said.

"I'm busy. You seem fine. Can it wait?" My terseness was in direct proportion to my pressure for meeting deadlines.

"Randi, get me a piece of paper and a pen." He said this firmly and I stopped touching all the electronics and grabbed the paper.

"Write this down: '*Your life is more than your job*.'" I wrote, as instructed, in big letters across the paper.

"Now, give me the paper," he said.

I handed him the paper and watched him scratch out his signature. It was clear the brain tumor was progressing because he struggled to write his name – Eugene V. Redmond. He handed me the paper, with his chicken-scratched signature, and we just looked at the paper and then at each other.

"Randi, you can do anything you want. *Make a difference, not an income*," he said. He pulled my hand toward him and we just hugged. I tucked the piece of paper away, a personal treasure that I cherish.

As the days progressed, he lost movement in his legs and we brought in a wheelchair. Then he needed assistance peeing. I know he was ashamed to have me hold the plastic jar for him, my strong capable father. By week seven, he was "shadowing," staying up all night and sleeping all day. He needed care 24/7. Between my husband, my mom and me we all did shifts. At night when my dad was awake, he'd insist that he was wet and every 10 minutes I'd have to dry off the phantom water. It was tougher than having an infant, at least they sleep a little. My husband and I were exhausted from staying up all night and working all day. We kept him home until we were unable to care for him, then we brought him to a lovely hospice with gardens outside and wood paneling in the rooms.

I visited every day. On the fifth day, the hospice nurse called our home, early in the morning, to report that my dad's breathing had changed, which was a sign that he was close to the end. I told my mom we'd go to the hospice and would not leave him; we'd pull an all-nighter if necessary and be with him through the end.

My mom and I arrived at the hospice and looked at him as he lay comfortably in bed without pain. The only movement in his body was his breathing at a constant rate, shallow and measured, like the second hand of a clock, steadily, predictably without any waiver of change. The predictable pattern gave my mom and me some comfort.

As the day wore on, my mom and I just sat in the room reading magazines and chatting, sometimes our reminiscing even made us laugh. I looked over at my dad at saw a slight smile. I think he liked hearing us talk. They say hearing is the last thing to go. I think he could tell we'd be fine together. My mom and I continued talking about decorating the family room to look like a picture she saw in a magazine. Time was easily passing, no drama, no pain. My father kept his breathing at a steady pace. Suddenly, I had this feeling. Nothing had changed in my father's breathing, nothing changed in his position, nothing changed in his facial expression, but I felt drawn to him. I walked over to him as he lay on the bed. "Mom, come here," I said.

"Why?" she asked, almost like she didn't want to get up from reading the magazine. She was growing comfortable with her new situation and the rhythm of the day.

"Just come here, now," I gently urged, wanting her to stay calm.

She put down the magazine, and got up from the chair and walked around the bed to see my father's face.

"Kiss him and tell him you love him."

"Now? Why?" she said.

"Just do it," I encouraged.

I kissed him first on his forehead and then my mom leaned down and kissed his cheek and said, "I love you."

He took one last inhale. Then he stopped breathing at that moment.

"What happened?" she asked, seeming a little confused.

I took my dad's hand and my mom's and just felt the moment and let my father lovingly pass. Deep down I do not believe my knowing the exact timing of when to say our final goodbye was a coincidence. I was overwhelmed with gratitude. Eugene Victor Redmond, my father, lived, and died, with dignity.

In the hospital room, listening to Gary's doctor, the words, "an excellent candidate for surgery" echo through my head as I try to pull myself together. I figure I have about 10 minutes of her time, max. I try to put her on the fast track to understanding my son and our family.

"Gary has a lot of choices ahead of him," I say. "You should know he is analytical and literal. He likes order and is very detailed. He thinks these traits and his experience with Crohn's disease will make him a good colorectal surgeon someday. So, he is not afraid of information. He'll need to have facts." She turns to Gary and says, "Oh, I am an analytic too. I like order. One time I turned around and drove home 45 minutes just to make sure I turned off the stove."

I'm not sure she gets what I am saying. I study her. I have no idea if she has kids or if she understands the personal turmoil our family is in. She reminds me of Steve's cousin Suzanne, a very bright woman who prides herself on being smart but seems to lack social IQ, maybe because she spent so much time with textbooks instead of friends. This doctor seems socially clueless, maybe because she is rushing. I continue to quickly try to get her to know me by using the elevator speech technique to make sure I hit the important highlights. It is the technique that says you are with the CEO in an elevator and you have three floors to get your message out to him. I keep this message simple. I only need one floor to make my point.

"Let me tell you about myself. I will ask lots of questions, *even the hard ones*, and I will push back to make sure we understand the options. I'll want to be involved and informed every step of the way."

She says, "Oh, you know when I started practicing I was offended by people asking me questions. But now I like the challenge."

The challenge? I was thinking we were on the same team. I am alarmed by her response but at least I know she got the message. She continues with, "Let's check the I.V." She walks over to the pump and looks at the medications. "It looks good. He'll be on the I.V.'s a couple of days. I'll be back tomorrow to check on him. He'll be fine for the rest of the day." As she races out the door, Gary's I.V. machine beeps. The machine is beeping loud, and it clearly is announcing that something needs to be done. Shouldn't she be concerned? But, the protocol train is in operation. Just like the engineer doesn't stop the train to collect tickets, because the conductor collects the tickets, the doctor knows it is protocol for someone else to stop the beeping. She doesn't look back.

After 10 minutes with the doctor, I am only slightly relieved that she thinks I.V. antibiotics will reduce Gary's pain, will kill off the infection and will reduce the swelling and make it easier to pee. That's my takeaway. I figure I'll wait to discuss the surgery with Gary's doctor, who is bound to show up sooner or later. With my nerves on edge from the outburst of the beeping, I hit the "concierge" button for help. In about five minutes a harried nurse comes in to fix the machine.

I still have to go back home to collect Gary's backpack and our family members, return to the hospital, and then go back home to sleep. I feel exhausted and drained and I start to wonder how I will find the energy for so many more trips in one day. But it's important to Gary to keep up with his school work and important to his brother to see that Gary is in a good place. It's important to me to keep everyone positive. It's not all about me, as a mom, I know it never is.

So, I drive home. I load Grandma and Matt into the car with the school supplies and drive back, just listening to music for the trip while Grandma and Matt sleep. They are still tired from the 2 a.m. hysterics with the emergency trip. I patiently walk Grandma to Gary's room. She cries less this time.

Gary shows off the flat panel TV and DVD player to his brother. Grandma remarks that Gary's spaghetti with meatball dinner looks yummy and she takes several bites. She must be getting used to the hospital because her appetite is back. I step outside the room to tell the nurse that I have a big meeting tomorrow at a university and I don't know what to do. I want to be with Gary but I am supposed to be presenting to 30 people and if they are interested in the long-term-care insurance employee benefit, I can actually generate some income. This is how I make money now.

After my dad died, I left the corporate world and decided to work for myself. I enjoy educating consumers on what is covered and not covered with medical insurance. Turns out, Medicare only pays if you can be rehabilitated. Once my dad turned down surgery, he was considered chronic and that is why they kicked us out. We paid for his subsequent medical needs.

Gary insists he'll be fine, but I need lots of assurance to leave him alone. The nurse explains he's just taking antibiotics through the I.V. to reduce the infection. There is nothing else happening. Gary will just be resting and waiting for the antibiotics to kick in. I should go to the meeting, she says. But I still haven't heard from his doctor and that surgery comment is haunting me.

I walk back into the room where Grandma is screaming, "Where's my pocketbook?" The kids are cracking up. This time I know she intentionally hid it just to get a rise out of them. It works and even I laugh. Gary assures me that he is not afraid of the hospital and tells me the call button for the nurses is his "concierge button." He wants to watch DVDs and rest and even finish the bio lab report. He does not need his mother tonight, he says. "I'll see you tomorrow," he says. "Good luck with your meeting."

I hug him tightly and try to sound strong and I promise to be back in the afternoon.

"Whenever, Mom," he says. "I've got my favorite DVDs, and all the time I want now."

What You Can Do Now

---

1. Ask the hard questions.

The doctors will answer only the questions you ask. The doctors would have removed a portion of my father's brain tumor and he might have lived an extra six months, but with pain and discomfort, which was not what he wanted.

2. Set expectations up front in your first meeting.

Tell the doctors how you want to work with them. Let them know if you want details and if you want to be involved in the decisions. Tell them about the personality of the patient and how they like to be handled. Be clear with your concerns.

3. Ignore the clock.

While in the hospital, you have nothing but time. If you get upset with how long it takes to get service you will be only raising your own stress level. Know that the hospital works quickly when it's a real emergency.

* * *

Chapter 5
Balanced and Battle-Ready

Back at home I can't sleep knowing that Gary is in the hospital. We still don't know what exactly is wrong with him. The new doctor is apparently calling the shots. I toss and turn through the night, praying for Gary's health, my strength and, in my big empty bed, job security for Steve. In just 48 hours my life seems to have turned upside down. The typical routine that my husband and I find security in has vanished. Steve is in New Jersey, Gary is in Hartford. I'm at home, listening to the second hand of my bedside clock. *Tick tock, tick tock, tick tock.* Time moves forward, steadily, predictably, as my mind races. I hear it tick and tock, until the morning alarm beeps at six.

I roll out of bed and into the shower. The thought of teaching strangers this morning instead of going to the hospital to be with Gary makes me feel ill. I place a small dab of shampoo into my palm. The clean scent does not wash away how awful I feel about going to work. Intellectually, I know Gary feels comfortable in the hospital and he does not physically need me present. I understand he is just hanging out as the I.V. drips antibiotics into his system, to "cool it off," as the doctor says. It is just a procedure that takes time. Everyone says I do not need to be there as the antibiotic drips and drops steadily into his system, until the machine beeps and signals it's done. But I want to be next to him. I want to be there as his thoughts fly as the antibiotics drip. I suspect Gary feels stuck in a place he doesn't want to be in. But I think he acts strong because he watches me act strong. He's seen me balance my husband's health issues, my mom's health issues and my full-time work to support the family. For better or for worse I'm a pro at holding back negative emotions, so the rest of my family can move forward – steadily, predictably. I don't know if all this acting is a good thing or a bad thing.

In the shower I think about postponing my presentation. But I know the last-minute cancellation will not go well with the head of human resources at the university. She has 30 people attending, even the provost. They want to learn about the employee benefit for long-term care insurance. She's worked hard to promote the session, and at any time she could replace me with someone more reliable. Plus, even if I get her to reschedule the session next month, it is the start of the holiday season, an automatic attendance reducer. In sales it's all about the numbers. The more prospects, the more potential business.

I take a deep breath, turn the water up to almost scalding and imagine Gary's pain. The water scorches my skin but I still can't get my pain level up to 12. I hit eight and see red blotches on my legs and feel them on my back before I turn down the scalding water and make myself stop. I think I'm going a little crazy. Gary will be watching DVD's, I rationalize. He's not even missing me. I know I'll be there in the early afternoon. I hope when I arrive, I'll hear the machine signaling that the drip is done.

So, I rinse my hair at a normal temperature, put on my corporate clothes and my high heels and drive to the session.

The university reserves a state-of-the-art appointed conference room for me. I like the wood paneling and boardroom feel. I realize it's a good thing I wore one of my best suits. I look like I fit in even though this is the last place I want to be. My presentation, stored on a thumb drive, easily loads onto the P.C. on the podium. I test the microphone and set up each of the armchairs with brochures. Looking over my handiwork, I am pleased with the perception of my life in control. I take a deep breath as I wait for the conference room to fill with attendees. With a couple of minutes before the session, I call

Gary on my cellphone, just to say good morning. He is energetic and he tells me he is in the middle of a movie. He sounds like he is doing better than I am. I am not sure whether I say, "I'll be there as soon as my presentation is over," for him or for me.

I feel so guilty about not being with Gary that I veer from my standard audience warm-up. Typically, I lead the audience with this question: "Who has cared for an elderly person?" Seeing the number of raised hands gives me a sense of how many people have been through the hardship of providing care to a loved one. In my business, there is a direct correlation to having provided care for someone and the likelihood of purchasing insurance. I also get a sense if a majority will understand when I tell the story of caring for my father. I feel that my personal experience differentiates me from someone just trying to make a sale.

In most of my seminars, I begin with the PowerPoint presentation. This time I don't even turn on the projector. I stand at the podium and tell them how I will be leaving right after the session to go back to the hospital to see my son, Gary. I can't believe I am telling them how he screams in pain. I tell them he has Crohn's disease. I am standing in front of an audience of strangers who came to hear about long-term care insurance and I divulge, probably sounding a little hysterical, how I don't know where Gary's doctor is. They stare at me and seem confused. Realizing I am totally off course, I stop saying anything. I just stare back. I think I have finally lost my mind. Then I see two people in the audience with their hands raised. I call on the first person, wondering if she is going to ask if I am going to talk about their new long-term care employee benefit. She says, "Randi, I have Crohn's." Before the woman can even finish her sentence, the other person bursts out, "I have it too!" I can't believe this. I never heard of this disease before Gary's initial diagnosis and now I discover it is so much more common than I'd ever thought. The first person continues, "Randi, after the presentation, if you have a second I'll talk to you. It's scary, but I cope." And the other person adds, "Me too."

They help snap me back into action. I thank them, turn on the projector, and ask, "How many of you have cared for an elderly person?" About half of the hands go up. The next 45 minutes, I am on my game, sharing stories, answering questions, hoping I am providing information that will make a difference in their lives. My father would be proud.

After the session, the two people with Crohn's quickly come up to me. One is a middle-aged female and the other is a middle-aged male. They both look fine, just thin. Not too thin, but sort of like they are masters at maintaining their weight. Before I knew the woman had Crohn's I might have envied her appearance because she seems so trim. I see a thin female and I never think it could be because she has a digestive disorder.

The woman says, "Randi, I take some medications and I'm fine. I've had some flare-ups but I'm able to live a productive life." I can't believe she's telling me this. I want to hug her. She continues, "It's scary because your son is so young, but they will figure out how to find a way for him to live without pain. I am a professor at the university and I haven't had to cancel a class in over a decade."

Before I can even respond, the gentleman says, "I just watch what I eat and I am on no medications. It took me a while to figure out the best foods for me, but I stick to it and I'm fine as well. I did have surgery over 20 years ago. I know how scary it is."

As they tell me their stories, I grasp this is a chronic disease, maybe a life sentence, but not necessarily a life-ender, like it was with Ruth's husband. The two people standing in front of me have solid careers at the university and families at home. They learned how to live with the disease. They confidently state the doctors will help Gary find a way to feel better, too. It is just a matter of time. I gratefully hug both of the attendees and pack up my things.

As I walk the long hallway out to my car, it occurs to me the doctors will treat Gary's physical symptoms. It is up to him – to us – to find role models so we can see how to navigate life's journey with this disease. The doctor gives a diagnosis. It is like the name of a destination to which you've never traveled. It's sort of like relocating. The doctor doesn't give you a travel brochure, filled with a description of a beautiful destination. Instead, he consistently warns you of the risks you may experience getting there. It's up to you to learn what the place really looks like and how to live there. As your journey starts, you might stare out the moving van window and see scenes that are horrifying. That's where I feel I am now on this trip, looking at a view of sick kids in a hospital. With only hearing doctors' disclaimers, it's hard for me to imagine Gary's journey ending beautifully.

I turn down the hall past oil portraits in ornate wooden frames of great university leaders and I realize that my morning excursion, which I was so reluctant to make, took me to a place where I could meet professionals with Crohn's who are married with children. I realize the two conference attendees are my travel brochure. They are the pictures of the beautiful places Gary can go. They are the gift I needed to calm me down about Gary and his future. My work today wasn't about an income after all. It was about connecting to people who could make a difference for us. I am grateful for this fork on my path.

Reaching my car, feeling some relief, I turn on the ignition and I call Gary. I feel so much better about the future and excited to tell Gary about the people I just met. But the way he says hello, I know something is wrong. It's only a two-syllable word, but I can hear volumes of anxiety in his voice. He tries to ask me about my meeting first, but I cut him off and I ask him what's wrong.

"The doctor put me on steroids, Mom," he says, each word getting lower and lower, as if he feels shame.

"What doctor?" I blurt out and feel my pulse start to race.

"The doctor from yesterday." His tone is deep and sad.

I know that Gary does not want to be on steroids. He's made this clear to Dr. Simmon, Gary's regular G.I., but Dr. Simmon is out of town, I've been told. Apparently, the 10-minute doctor is either unaware or doesn't care. When Gary was first diagnosed with Crohn's and had the choice of either taking steroids or not eating solids for a month, his symptoms revealed a moderate case of Crohn's. Gary researched steroids and came to pretty much the same conclusion as what he found on the website www.ehealthmd.com. Here's what it says:

"Steroids are powerful, potentially toxic drugs that reduce inflammation and suppress the body's immune system. Prednisone and prednisolone are the most commonly used steroids for treatment of Crohn's disease and ulcerative colitis... While they are very useful, steroids can produce a number of side effects ranging from annoying to dangerous.

• Annoying side effects include puffiness in the face, acne, insomnia, tremors, night sweats, weight gain, and mood disturbances.

• Dangerous side effects include increased blood pressure, osteoporosis, severe depression, and even psychosis. Long-term steroid use can cause cataracts and glaucoma." [1]

Not surprisingly, Gary chose nutritional therapy to avoid steroids. Gary told me he did not want a moon face, acne and the possible side effect of anxiety. He wanted to look and feel like everybody else. Every day for a month, he popped open eight cans of Ensure or Boost and drank it for breakfast, lunch and dinner, even at school. To show support on Tuesday nights we all sat around the table and drank Ensure or Boost for dinner, even Grandma. (Although after dinner when Gary went to bed, she'd sneak chocolate chip cookies and milk.) Gary achieved the same results the steroids would deliver but without the side effects: At the end of the month, Gary's digestive system was stabilized and his diarrhea and cramps were minimized. He was given the choice to keep with the nutritional therapy three times a year to try to remain in remission or to take Pentasa, a mild medication. Nutritional therapy was so tough he chose 12 Pentasa pills a day. But he never took a steroid. Now, I think the steroids are to reduce the inflammation from his bladder infection, which causes pain during urination. Same drug, for a different purpose, but Gary would rather live with the pain until surgery, which will fix the problem.

On my cellphone, I ask Gary, "Did you ask any questions?" I know my tone sounds blameful, but I'm so shocked, I can't help myself.

"Yeah. She said I might get depressed or happy, but it will help with the pain. She just told me to take it. I feel bad, Mom. I didn't want to take them but I didn't have a choice." He sounds like he feels violated.

"You did nothing wrong, Gary. If you need steroids, I'm sure there is a good medical reason." I look at my GPS, which estimates arrival time of 40 minutes. I say, "I'll be there in half an hour. I'll speak to her. Don't worry." I try to strike a reassuring tone, but fear I failed.

When I hang up, I really understand the expression "My blood is boiling." I am livid. How could the doctor put Gary on the medication when his G.I. knew Gary didn't want steroids? Gary told her he didn't want steroids when I told her, clearly, that I wanted to be involved every step of the way.

I speed on I-91 and zip into the hospital parking garage. I just want to jump out of the car and dash to Gary. However, I have to find a parking space first. I circle the first floor and find no spots. I end up behind another car searching for a spot. A man, who looks like someone's grandpa, is in a big old gray dinged-up Cadillac in front of me. He maneuvers cautiously to look for his spot. I crawl behind him to the second floor and still no spots, for either of us. We circle the third floor and he still does not find a spot. I bet this is how road rage starts. I actually imagine blowing up his car just to be able to park first. Finally, on the fourth level, after 20 prolonged minutes of searching, he advances his vehicle into a spot. With him no longer in front of me, I floor it to the fifth floor and I accelerate between the white lines of the first empty spot I see. I brake fast and hard to avoid hitting the garage wall. My driving feels like my emotions, barely in control. Wanting to make up for lost time, I sprint to the hospital entrance by going down the five flights of stairs, in high heels, instead of taking the elevator. I huff and puff my way to the security guard at the hospital's entrance. I'm behind three people all checking in to get a sticker for visiting. It forces me to slow down and catch my breath. I tell the guard my name, wait for the printer to release my sticker and rip off the backing and place the sticky side on my violet silk blouse. I regain speed and race through the halls to the elevator up to the sixth floor. I bolt out of the elevator and rush to the nurses' station. I am huffing and puffing again. I feel like a pressure cooker ready to lose its top.

"Where is Gary's doctor from yesterday?" I think I sound calm, but probably my loud request and breathlessness is a dead giveaway that I am upset. I bet I don't look great either.

"We can page her if you'd like. Why do you want to speak with her?" someone at the nurses' station says to me in an artificial-sweetener-laced voice.

"My son is on steroids and no one called me."

I don't wait for a response and burst into Gary's room. He's not reading. He's not watching DVDs. He is staring into space. "Mom, they put me on steroids. I screwed up."

"You did nothing wrong, Gary. I've asked to speak to the doctor. It could be you needed the steroids. We'll find out."

I fear it will be hours before the doctor arrives. I know that we are just another family and they are busy. I sit on the side of the bed and take Gary's hand in mine. I like the feeling of the warmth of his hand. It feels real. It helps me regain my grounding. I decide to make this a teachable moment for Gary. I can't believe how many teachable moments this kid is getting. I really wish he was in school learning basic biology and not doctor-patient relations through me, but this our reality and we have to accept it.

"Gary, here's the trick: If when the doctor comes in and I am hysterical and yell 'how come you put him on steroids without consulting me first?' I will lose the argument."

He looks at me.

"You see, Gary, if I yell and scream like I feel I want to, the doctor will see a hysterical woman and I will lose credibility. I'll be another crazy, emotional, overprotective mom. She'll tell me about medical protocol, all the reasons steroids are needed and use fancy medical lingo that I do not understand, so I can't object. She'll be professional, knowledgeable and objective; clearly a better disposition for decision-making. So the trick is to stay calm, even though I want to scream at her for not calling me first. Make sense?" I look at him to see if he is paying attention and he nods.

"So," I continue, "I'll ask her, acting very composed, a series of questions. I'll make them easy and friendly to get her off guard. Then, I'll nail her with the process question about how our family requested to work with her." In my GE training, not meeting customer expectations was considered a defect. All I want is to understand why she implemented this without our consent and why he's on steroids. And I need her to acknowledge her mistake.

Gary seems skeptical. "No way, Mom. The doctor is going to apologize to you and take me off the steroids?" I am his mother, not a superhero.

"Well, if we're convinced steroids are the best course of action, Gary, you will need to take them. But, you will understand why. OK?" I try to sound confident, like I'll be back in control soon. I feel like I am back in the office. I am so used to office politics that this conflict feels familiar to me. Being in well-known territory allows me to feel some strength return. I survived 18 years of layoffs at GE in part because I am a master at this proven technique: Find solutions that improve team performance.

We sit quietly for a few seconds and our tender moment is unexpectedly interrupted with three rapid knocks on the door.

The doctor enters with a troubled look on her face. The room is small and before she even sits down on the chair next to the desk, I see three more people enter the room. I never have seen these people in my life. They are all men ranging in age from 30 to 50, wearing ties. I can't tell if they are doctors, lawyers or the CEO of the hospital. No one introduces himself. My pulse races. I feel sweaty. The last person to squeeze into the room is Gary's nurse. She goes directly to his side.

I thought the doctor and I would share a private conversation, but clearly she needs backup. I feel intimidated with all these people in the room. It reminds me of GE operation review sessions – impersonal, battle-ready, with the higher-ups looking for the weak link. It was a requirement of Jack Welch, the CEO of GE during my tenure, to eliminate 10 percent of the workforce every year. His rationale was to keep only the top performers. At this rate, after five years, over 50 percent of the workforce turns over. Another reason I survived 18 years of "rightsizing" is because I understood another basic concept: *Barracudas prey only on the weak.* I learned how to get the other person to look weak by making them either become defensive or apologize. It was heart-aching and excruciating and absolutely necessary to my corporate survival.

I need to pull myself together. I mentally put on my battle armor and get up from the bed and move to sit, alone, on the couch. I sit up straight to be the same height as the doctor, who is sitting by the desk. I look at the men directly as they huddle together in the corner. I take a deep breath.

"You have a question?" the 10-minute doctor inquires.

"Yes," I say, forcing myself to smile. "Before we get started, I'm not even sure I know your name." I say this first to show the "audience" she brought with her that she and I have no relationship. Also, this is the start of the process of me gaining control. She's answering to me.

"Oh, I'm Dr. Diane Stark." She says this tenderly and I assume she adds her first name to seem more personal.

"OK, well, yesterday we met for about 10 minutes and I made sure to tell you about my son and myself." I establish the fact that her encounter with Gary was brief. "Can you tell me what I told you about my son?"

"Yes," she enthusiastically answers. She is a doctor and I know from Steve's cousin that they like to look smart. She proudly repeats, "He's an analytic and wants information. That's why I told him about the steroids and gave him a chance to ask questions."

"Good." I confirm to her audience that she got the answer right by looking up at them and nodding my head. She, too, looks over her shoulder at her audience and smiles. It's almost like a game show. I continue with round two. "And what did I tell you about myself?"

"Gary had an inflammation in his intestine causing him pain. The antibiotics will not reduce the inflammation. It is medical protocol to use steroids." She doesn't answer my question. But at least I know what the steroids are for. Apparently it's not for his bladder. She adds in more medical terminology that seems to get the audience shaking their heads in agreement with her decision.

I speak up. "I am not saying I disagree with your medical decision. That was not my question," I say firmly. At this point, I look over at Gary and he appears to be sleeping. I think he pretends because he is mortified. This is the doctor who said she'd bring him the trilogy of the *"Lord of the Rings"* on DVD and he doesn't want her pissed off.

The doctor ignores my comment. She continues her explanation about reducing inflammation in what sounds like medical mumbo jumbo to me. The whole room seems to be on the protocol train. Even the nurse is nodding her head in agreement with the people in the back of the room. I seem to be the only reluctant passenger. I interrupt her. "What did I tell you about myself?"

"That you'd want to be involved in understanding his care," she admits.

"Yes," I say, again looking over at the audience and nodding my head so they know she got the answer right. "So, at 11 a.m. you gave him steroids, correct?"

"Yes," a firm answer.

"Did you call my cellphone?" the answer of which, I already knew. There were no messages on my phone.

"No," still said firmly, but softer.

"Did you call my home?" I say it soft too, mirroring her tone. I don't want to be perceived as a mean bitch.

"No." She adjusts herself in the chair and doesn't look back.

"So, you did not make any effort to contact me? Was this a medical emergency that couldn't wait until you could speak to me today? It's 3 p.m. now." I know it's like re-stabbing the point, but I need to make sure these people learn how to most effectively work with my family. I am not blindly going down a path I do not understand. I need to ensure that this will not happen again.

"No," she says.

I continue with the line of questioning. "OK, well, did you call his pediatrician?" I ask in my normal voice.

She doesn't say "no" this time. She looks up at me with a troubled look on her face and then turns to the back of the room and states in defense of her actions, "I spoke to Gary's G.I. and her partner, Dr. Hughes. I did not make this decision in isolation."

She stares at me. "No, I did not contact you. I'm sorry. I did what we always do. Dr. Simmon told me you had an issue with steroids but he saw the pros and cons of administering them. Dr. Hughes and I agreed it was the best course of action."

She apologizes, like I told Gary she would. He does not peek out from under his sheet, but I have a strong feeling he listens to every word. I can see she is not happy to have made a mistake, but I gain much more respect for her to admit it in front of her colleagues, especially so fast.

I win the first point in this battle. I am grateful to have learned this power technique. The one where the aggressor (me) uses "I – You" language to make the other person (the doctor) squirm. I hated when it was done to me. The recipient either gets defensive or apologizes. Like in sports, when somebody is on the defensive all the time, it's hard to win. I am gaining some control. It feels good.

"I am not disagreeing with your medical decision," I say, "I just don't understand it yet. If Dr. Simmon has pros and cons we want to understand them. The same way I didn't even know your name is the same way I have never even met Dr. Hughes."

"Oh, he's the leading pediatric Crohn's doctor." Status does not impress me. She reminds me of Steve's cousin, again. His cousin values titles and possessions and is so competitive that she judges others by their clothes and cars. She was valedictorian of her high school class and knows she is smarter than most people. So she rarely feels she can learn from others. She's condescending. I take this statement in the same way.

"I've never met him and he's never seen my child," I say. "I'd like to speak to my doctor first before we make this decision." The room is silent. All eyes are on me. I take a deep breath before I ask my next question.

"Is it life-threatening?" I ask.

"No," she states.

"So he's off the steroids until I speak to Dr. Simmon." I don't phase it as a question.

"I am so sorry," she says again, like it's a line in a script, sounding like she's on the software help desk in India. It sounds sincere the first time you hear it but after multiple calls to the help desk you realize it is part of the training. "I'd hate for Gary to have to come off of standard medical protocol because I made a mistake by not calling you," she says. "Now he has to be in pain because of your decision." Ouch! She's trying for a comeback. She is a fighter. She's not using any GE technique here, but a tougher one: guilt. But with a Jewish mother from the Bronx, I've trained for this all my life.

I know this is not some kind of mind game. I know that my child is in excruciating pain when he urinates. How can I be so callous as to let my son be in such pain if it can be reduced? The thing is, he's scheduled for surgery in four days. Apparently the surgeon plans to cut out the diseased intestine and the mass of fluids by Gary's bladder in the hope of eliminating Gary's pain. If he starts steroids, won't he need to be weaned off of them before the surgery? I have no idea how long they expect him to be on them, because no one discusses it with me. No one even told us how long it takes for the steroids to work. We never even got the chance to ask the hard questions. Are the risks better than the pain? I don't know any of these answers.

"He is off the steroids until I speak to Dr. Simmon and my questions are answered. Kindly have him call me," I say to the doctor and to the men in suits. I'm not done, though. Now that I've won both points I can be more gracious. "Let me explain," I say. "You've been on this path before and this is our first time. We feel like we're in the forest and don't know where to go. So instead of us feeling lost, I am sure you have brochures or information about the disease. Like what we can expect. So everything is not a surprise." I throw this out for two reasons. I figure she has some documentation on the disease and it gives her an opportunity to end on a positive note by saying she'll accept the action item. I also want to see if she will follow through on bringing in the information.

"I can bring you some information in the morning. Just know every case is different," she says. She seems grateful to be able to have something positive to offer. Dr. Stark goes over to Gary. She taps on his shoulder and Gary pulls his head out from under the sheet. She apologizes and says she'll bring the *"Lord of the Rings"* trilogy in for him to watch, tomorrow. Gary smiles like he won on every count. Just as fast as the mystery men entered, they leave the room ... without even shaking my hand. Dr. Stark leaves with them.

Gary seems thrilled to be off the steroids until Dr. Simmon answers our questions. He reaches for the remote control and zaps through stations. I go to my laptop. A quick Google search confirms my suspicion: The wrong drugs could hurt my son. At least 1.5 million people are harmed every year from errors with medications. One study indicates that 400,000 preventable drug-related injuries occur in hospitals each year.[2] That's what I'm discovering on my laptop in the hospital.

If I'm going to be honest, I think that's what happened to my son to begin with. I partly blame myself for Gary's disease. I was on a business trip when Gary was five years old and he was sick with a raging temperature. My husband called me and said Gary had a 105-degree fever and his eye was swollen almost shut. Steve took Gary to the pediatrician but she wasn't there that day. Her physician's assistant diagnosed Gary with cellulitis, a very serious infection, and started him on double doses of Rocephin, a powerful antibiotic, injected into his backside for five days in a row. Steve took Gary for the series of double injections. The doctor confirmed the physician's assistant's diagnosis to Steve. I was traveling. I trusted everyone and did not ask any questions; I was too busy on an acquisition. When I returned, Gary was better, so the doctor's treatment for the cellulitis seemed valid. I did not observe any side effects and I was grateful. The doctor followed medical protocol. She cured him of cellulitis. She saved his eyesight. But I always wondered if a kindergartener really needed five days of double injections of such a strong antibiotic.

I found a study originally published in German entitled, "Crohn's disease caused by antibiotics? A medical hypothesis based on epidemiologic data."[3] Ludwig Demling notes that "increasing incidence of Crohn's disease over the last 50 years has paralleled the growing use of antibiotics in human and veterinary medicine." He claims "antibiotics can induce in bacteria a capability for producing toxins. Statistical considerations also indicate that prior antibiotic treatment promotes the development of Crohn's disease. It seems logical to assume that, in persons with a relevant genetic predisposition, this disease is caused by intestinal bacteria, the biological (not morphological) properties of which have been modified by antibiotics." These findings substantiated my gut instinct. I looked for another study and found one from the University of Nottingham.[4]

I am an engineer, not a biologist, but it looked like they used valid methods for the study.

"A total of 587 Crohn's disease cases and 1460 controls were available for analysis. We found that antibiotic use 2-5 years pre-diagnosis occurred in 71 percent of cases compared with 58 percent of controls."[5] Even though their summary had more technical terms, it was the conclusion in the abstract that said it all to me. "We found a statistically significant association between Crohn's disease and prior antibiotic use."[6] I believe the trigger for Gary may have been the aggressive use of antibiotics. I may be wrong. I found a limited scientific backup for my hypothesis but my hypothesis is that the antibiotics changed Gary's gut flora balance. The gut flora are the good and bad bacteria in the intestine. The antibiotics do not discriminate. They kill everything. My hypothesis is that when Gary completed the antibiotics, the bad bacteria grew back faster than the good bacteria. The bad bacteria without the good bacteria to counteract them attacked his intestines.

I haven't found a doctor in the United States who believes there is documented evidence that the antibiotics contributed to the problem and I agree that not everyone who takes antibiotics gets Crohn's, thankfully. But, antibiotics do change the gut flora levels. I bet massive antibiotics like Gary was given really impacted his intestinal balance. No one mentioned he should eat yogurt or take a probiotic to balance out his system at the time. To me, Gary ended up with the disease because he has a genetic disposition, experienced an environmental event with the massive doses of antibiotics and lacked the appropriate nutrition to help curtail the disease.

Six years later we were back in Gary's pediatrician's office. Gary had severe cramps and diarrhea and the protocol train started up again to treat these new symptoms. I watched a whole new battery of tests being administered, concluding with a diagnosis of Crohn's. As Gary went from one emergency room to another, one doctor's office to another, they repeated the same tests. Sometimes, they'd ask for copies of records, but for the most part it seemed as if new tests were given with no regard for the radiation levels being administered for the CT scans, the X-rays, the M.R.I.'s between locations.

I came to this realization: No one was tracking the effects of these tests. The impact of these tests and treatments may be years away. Just like I believe the impact of all those antibiotics was years away and finally presented as Crohn's. As Gary grows up and continues to need medical support for his disease, he'll have doctors who will say, "Oh, this new symptom is a consequence of a previous treatment." The new doctor will follow the protocol for that new symptom. Gary is too naïve to understand the big picture right now. He just wants to trust today's doctor; he wants his pain to go away now. I realize that if I don't map out the entire journey, he might end up on a very dangerous path.

Four years later here we go again. This time it's with steroids, another medication, with known side effects. Only this time, there is not an immediate threat, like it was to save his eyesight. It is to help him cope with four more days of pain, until surgery. My friend Ruth said her husband's problems started with the steroids. To me, steroids are like cigarettes – a starter drug.

Gary flips through the TV stations and my cellphone rings. It's Dr. Simmon. I'm thrilled to hear his voice but I hear lots of voices in the background. I figure he's in a hall on a conference break. Instead of bombarding him with questions, I let him talk; I know his time is limited. He apologizes for being away and says that his partner, Dr. Stark, has apprised him of the situation.

"I'll be free at 7 p.m. I'll call you then to discuss the pros and cons of the steroids," he says firmly and hangs up.

Finally I'll be able to speak with Dr. Simmon! He knows me. He knows Gary. He knows Gary's history firsthand. I figure I won't wait in the hospital for the call because then I'll get home too late. I want to be home at a decent time so I can spend some quality time with Matt. I keep hearing my mom in the background on the phone when I speak to Matt. "Bring in the mail! Bring up the laundry! Get me the scissors!" she's saying. I sense my mother's topsy-turvy life without our usual routines is stressing her out, so she is screaming even more. Matt is the only one home and the recipient of her continual demands. She says she still is independent, but she doesn't seem to realize she is totally dependent on us to help her get her stuff done. It's out of love and respect, but we spend our days jumping around the house at her command.

Matt doesn't say it but I know he needs a hug. I know I would need one if I were there alone. I decide to leave the hospital at 6:30 p.m. This way I can talk to the doctor while driving and still be home at a reasonable hour. I think through my concerns to prepare for the phone call. Maybe there are good reasons to take steroids four days before surgery? Maybe Gary won't need them too long? Maybe I am wrong and steroids work instantly to relieve the pain and will not take a couple of days to kick in? Maybe Dr. Stark is right. I just want Dr. Simmon's opinion.

I leave the hospital and notice that most of the leaves have already fallen off the trees. The 40-degree temperature and damp rain give me the same chill on the outside that I feel on the inside. I enter my car and turn up the heat, and within a couple of minutes I pull onto I-91 southbound. The warmth embraces me, comforts me and frees me to release my pent-up emotions. The tears start to flow. I'm raw with fear and sadness. I grip the steering wheel.

As I drive to keep up with traffic, the windshield wipers cannot work fast enough to keep up with the rain. I can barely see out the window. I try to focus on the road and to think about my questions for Dr. Simmon. I want to understand the purpose of the antibiotics versus the steroids.

At exactly 7 p.m. my cellphone rings. I reach to the cup holder next to me to grab it and flip it open. As I look for the little phone button to press for the speaker feature, so I can have a hands-free call, my car swerves. I hear the brakes screech on the car behind me.

Then I hear another car slam on its brakes. I do not hear any crashes. I do not look back. I just want to speak to Dr. Simmon.

"Randi, Dr. Simmon here." He sounds faint.

"Yes."

"I'm on a flight and we are in the process of taking off. I have less than five minutes to talk. I know that isn't a lot of time. I want you to know that this is not a private place so the person next to me can hear what we are discussing. Are you OK with that?"

"Yes." Like I really care about privacy now. But I know it's HIPAA rules that require patient privacy and he feels obligated to follow all the regulations of the law. Clearly, we're on the protocol train, again.

"I spoke to Dr. Stark today and I understand your concerns about steroids. I know you never met her before but she is my partner and I support her medical decision." He blurts this out, stating his position so clearly, that even with a bad connection I hear him sharp. The tone in his voice seems like he is concerned about keeping a unified medical front, not about my son.

Instantly, I feel this lump in my throat. He's Gary's doctor, but she is his partner. Apparently he is going to support her. I know he'll side with her because otherwise it will mean she did something medically wrong. But I still want answers to my questions. At least I want to know the risks of this path and why it is a needed step. As I pick up the phone so he can hear me better when I speak, my car swerves again. This time I don't hear any brakes slamming down behind me.

I ask, "What do the steroids do?"

Dr. Simmon starts to answer the question but he is interrupted by the stewardess who is addressing the passengers about the overhead compartment. She is giving the safety speech about air pressure and placing the cups over your mouth. We all know the speech. It takes at least three minutes. We can't hear each other while she is speaking and I realize that I am not going to get the information I need to understand why my son has to take steroids.

The second she stops, Dr. Simmon says, "Randi, the plane is leaving in one minute."

I panic inside. Do I just give in and trust their experience? Or do I hold my ground, so I can make an informed decision?

Before my father died, the little girl in me would just do what the doctors said. But I've come so far as a woman, I realize I don't know the risks of the steroids, how long they will take to work and the outcomes. I still have too many questions. I would never have one of my clients take an insurance policy without a thorough meeting to understand it. Now, I'm expected to have less than a three-minute conversation and commit my child to a course of action with known negative side effects? With an insurance policy, you get a 30-day free look period and if you cancel there are no lasting repercussions. Pressure tactics are frowned upon. But perhaps not with doctors. I never purchase anything feeling unsure. So, I go with my instincts.

"Doctor, Gary is not to have steroids until I understand the justification for taking them. Stop them immediately." I say it strong, clear and probably even the person next to Dr. Simmon on the plane hears me as well.

"OK." He hangs up.

I drive home. It is an eerie feeling to tell the doctors what to do. It makes me even more aware that I need to ask questions. Maybe if I'd done that when Gary was five, I'd know about gut flora and the need for the probiotic. I never asked, they never told me. We just blindly followed the path. Now, I understand that the doctors follow protocol because it is safer. They use years of medical research and testing to back up their decisions. They can tell you the probabilities of outcomes by disclosing the risks. This helps prevent lawsuits and justification if there is a lawsuit. So, by recommending a process with predictable negative medical outcomes I sense they are more comfortable taking a risky path than an unknown path.

To me, there seems to be a conflict of interest: many research studies are paid for by the companies that sell the drugs. The people providing the medical justifications are selling the doctors their products. Therefore, I need to make sure their recommendations are truly best for one patient in particular, my son Gary.

I call Gary and tell him the news. "You are off the steroids, until someone explains them to us."

"Mom, I don't think I need them. I can live with this pain for four more days."

I arrive home and turn on the light to the garage. I might be living in a house of cards but right now I feel like a superhero. I did exactly what I said I would for Gary. I go upstairs and hug Matt. I actually sleep soundly for the first time in two nights.

When I get to the hospital the next day, Dr. Stark is talking to my son. Gary is smiling. As I approach his bed, he holds up the trilogy of "*Lord of the Rings*."

"Good morning," she says to me, as if she swallowed the same artificial sweetener as the nurse at the station.

"Good morning," I say, as if I drank the same cup of laced coffee.

"I spoke with Dr. Hughes and Dr. Simmon and since Gary is going to have surgery in three days and he can withstand the pain, he doesn't need steroids. We will not be giving them to him," she states.

Now I am *really* skeptical. How come he doesn't even need them? I was prepared to ask questions and change positions if necessary. I look at Dr. Stark. Her eyes are tired. I guess last night was tough on her. She probably had to admit a mistake in front of those people, whoever they were. It was basic patient relations that she screwed up. They can't talk medical mumbo jumbo to cover up mistakes about showing basic respect for families.

"Here is some background information for you on Crohn's. I hope it helps," she says, handing me pages and pages from a medical journal, the kind in small print with black and white body-part diagrams. I look down and know the technical information looks like it's beyond my layman's understanding, but as I take the papers, I see the human side of her and I'm genuinely appreciative. I give her a hug and say, "Thank you."

She holds me tighter than I expect. Like the hug is something she really needs. She beams as if I gave her an "A" on the final. I get the sense that my small act of compassion is a big deal. "You see, Gary, grownups can learn from their mistakes," she says directly to him. "We can have frank discussions and still move forward."

She seems proud to make it a teachable moment for Gary. I feel very moved and I hope Gary doesn't roll his eyes. She says, "Steroids can cause complications in surgery. It's better to have the surgery without them if possible."

Really?

Gary smiles so broad that I see all his beautiful teeth shine. I'm smiling, too. Even though I am not educated in the medical field I was able to make the right call for my son.

Things seem to change in the hospital from this point. Gary's nurse seems a little afraid of us. She starts explaining every single thing she is doing. "Now I am touching this button," she says, going into detail. Clearly, they must have written in Gary's records that we are to be made aware of everything and given the opportunity to ask questions. It's sort of nerve-wracking to hear all this detail from everyone who enters the room to care for Gary, but to me it is better than being clueless.

Now these strangers understand how we operate as a family, on information. I understand they have a well-oiled machine they work in everyday. They move through the machine gears ducking and turning in synchronization with each other, sometimes forgetting that a newcomer might be terrified. I think they believe that trust in the machine is essential. After all, they know they are the experts. Yet, for me questions abound. They don't know it, but I am an electrical engineer by training and I want to know, what does this part do? How does this work? Where is this process going? Why do we need to take this step? Who is controlling the process? Everyone says ask questions, but I feel as if the machine slows down for them when I try to get up to speed. I see their frustration creep up. They have other people to process.

The doctors are the first to say they do not have all the answers. I realize maybe that's why they don't like the questions. But this experience reinforces my resolve: Unless it's life-threatening, I must STOP the machine and understand exactly what is happening. I'm incorporating these new people onto OUR team.

What You Can Do Now

---

1. Talk to others with the disease. Listen to their story.

The doctors are responsible for your physical care. It is up to us to find role models so we can see how to navigate life's journey with a disease.

2. Ask WHY, say NO.

Even if you have no idea what they are talking about, ask "Why?" You will get a sense of their conviction. If you have any doubt about a procedure or a medication say "No" until you are comfortable.

3. If something goes wrong, do not yell at the doctor.

You will lose credibility. Stay calm. Ask for a meeting. Point out where you feel they missed your expectations and be clear that it is not to happen again. I only had 10 minutes with my initial meeting with Dr. Stark, but I was clear I wanted to be involved in every non-emergency medical decision. When she put my son on steroids, without consulting me, she had to admit her mistake, could not say I was being overdramatic, and the hospital documented that every person we came in contact with was to meet our expectations by explaining what they were doing and why.

* * *

Chapter 6
Operations in the Hospital

Gary is receiving a cocktail of four antibiotics. The doctors said the names so fast, I'm not sure what the drugs are called. I cringe with each drip into his system. The doctors repeatedly tell me the antibiotics are necessary. They will make him better, although I don't exactly understand why or how. It seems to me they are trying to fix his bladder problem with the same type of medicine that I think caused the Crohn's. But what do I know? I'm a tired mom. In corporate America, I learned, repeated complaining doesn't help. It's perceived as whining. Whiners are weak. You want to be heard? Come up with a better idea. I don't have one. Therefore, I am resigned to the fact that they are the experts.

I settle in to what I expect will be three monotonous days until the big surgery day. There is a rhythm, a pace, a beat, a predictability here that I was too overwhelmed to notice upon Gary's admittance. I start to recognize people. I can now tell the housekeeping person from the nurse. I know a P.C.A. from a doctor. Meals are delivered at same time every day. Gary watches the full *"Lord of the Rings"* trilogy twice. That's about 20 hours of DVD pleasure. In between, he takes bathroom breaks and screams until he fully relieves himself. The screams have become part of his process.

It's hard for me to sit and wait and I have no interest in *"Lord of the Rings."* I'm used to being productive. I feel I need a purpose, a direction, otherwise, my thoughts will race out of control. I'm afraid I'll get frustrated and, like my mother, I'll start screaming and barking orders at everybody. In addition to my electrical engineering degree, I have an MBA from Boston University. In the MBA program, I studied operations and trained to find process improvements. This is what I'm good at. I loved studying processes. OK, maybe obsessed is a more accurate description. Since I need a role here, or I'm going to lose it, I know what I'll do. I'll use this free time to write down everything happening in the hospital, to see if I can help improve the process.

Patient relations seems to be a good place to start. In the room with "*Lord of the Rings*" blaring, I challenge myself to help find a way to improve standard protocol for how they deal with our family. As each person enters the room and sees me diligently typing on my laptop, I tell them I am keeping a journal of our experience, that it is fascinating to me and that I hope one day to share it with others. In addition to keeping a journal, I decide to implement a tool my father used when he was in the hospital. It was a list of people involved in his care. Privately, he called it his "shit list." He's a former Navy guy. If you screwed up, he tracked it. He kept the list next to his bedside. When someone came in, he had the worker write down his or her name. When the individual did a wonderful job he drew a star next to the name. My dad found a way to motivate workers to go the extra mile for him. It became routine for the care providers to glance at the list for their co-workers' names to see if everyone was doing their best job. They raised each other's performance bar. My dad received amazing care before they threw him out. My system will be similar to his. I grab a piece of paper on the desk and write out some columns – Date, Name, Position, Results – at the top of the page.

Then I go back to typing about my conversation with Dr. Simmon from the plane. A trim woman in her 50's, who looks in shape from pushing the heavy cleaning cart constantly, enters the room. She goes right to the trash can and starts to empty it.

"Hi, what's your name?" I ask.

"Marta," she says. She looks at me strangely like I'm not supposed to talk to her.

"Great, Marta. Gary is going to be here awhile. I've seen you before. Nice to see you again." She looks at me quizzically. I decide she can't be any more confused by this interaction. So, I make her the first person to hear about the list. I get up from the couch and walk over to the desk and pick up the piece of paper.

"You are doing an excellent job keeping this room clean, Marta. I want to be able to thank everyone who helps Gary at the end of his stay. I plan on writing a letter to the CEO, telling him about the wonderful care Gary receives. Will you write your name on the piece of paper and your role? "

"Sure."

She seems a little afraid of me. I suspect she's been told to answer my questions. Next to her name, Marta Bazin, she writes Environmental Services and says in a heavy accent, "I think this is a good idea. I see a lot here. You know, nobody ever wrote to my boss about me doing a good job. There is a lot to do." She wipes down the sink as she talks.

"How unfortunate," I say in a sympathetic tone.

"You know," she says wiping down the countertop. "You seem like a nice family. I see you go home at night... When your son has his operation, I think you should stay."

She is the first person to say this to me.

"Really?" I was planning to stay over, but not because I thought it was necessary. I wonder why she thinks I need to stay?

Marta continued, "All I'll say is if you love someone, you'd be with them here. Like I said, I see a lot." She doesn't say anything else and moves to the bathroom, where I don't follow her to continue the conversation. After she finishes her job, I tell her, "This room is spotless. Thank you so much." She sees me put a star next to her name.

"Thanks. See you tomorrow!" she says.

Now that I have a purpose, I type fast, documenting all my interactions with Dr. Stark and how Dr. Simmon called me from the plane. I am feeling productive again during these endless hours of waiting. Because I am working, I have a small sense of normalcy. I even like how the environment has changed since our first day here. The formerly stark impersonal room is filled with balloons, stuffed animals and cards from Gary's friends and family. There actually is no more room for another teddy bear or even a small balloon on the window sill. As my fingers eagerly type, a delivery man breaks the rhythm of my keystrokes with another special delivery. I look up and Gary tells the delivery man to place the white teddy bear on the desk. Gary thanks the man.

Gary says, "People care about me, Mom. Look at this room!"

When the non-stop calls came in the first day and everyone asked, "What can I do to help?" my standard response was for them to send a card or a balloon. Now, not only does Gary see that he really matters to others, all who enter Gary's room can see the support we have in our community.

When I take breaks from writing and walk the halls, my heart sinks when a child is in a sterile room with no balloons or cards. With a little detective work, I discover it's mostly repeat patients in rooms with the barren walls. To me it sends a strong signal that either the child and the family are alone or that the hospitalization is so common, it's not worth trying to brighten the dark circumstances. I hope we never get to that point.

With my process-improvement mentality in the forefront of my mind, I venture out of the room on a discovery expedition. First stop, the nurses' station. It is smack in the center of the floor. Across from the nurses' station is an electronic board with all the patients listed, first name only, and the room number. Next to the room number is the name of a nurse assigned. As I glance at the big white board with patients, the only thing I care about is how many patients are on the floor for the day, because my operations mindset figures the fewer patients, the more time the nurses have to focus on Gary and their other assigned cases.

I've noticed the nurses are on their feet for most of their shift, moving rapidly from room to room. One of their main functions appears to be monitoring medications. Gary has four bags of I.V. fluids dripping into him at the same time. When one medicine bag is empty the machine beeps. The nurses race to his room to add medications and stop the beeping. As I walk the floor, I hear machines constantly beep from room to room. I watch the nurses in constant pursuit, moving in multiple directions to turn them off. It's sort of like the nurses play a game of Beat the Clock. They run around trying to add medications before the machine beeps, but mostly the medications run out first and the machine wins. Many times, the nurses are so busy the machine gets to sing its glory for a full five minutes before the harried nurse comes in to turn it off and start the next round of the game. Since the beeping is irritating to hear, typically the patients hit their "concierge button" for the nurse to come to their room, just to turn off the machine. So, maybe the nurse prioritizes where to go by which patient seems most aggravated. I calculate, if each nurse has eight patients, which seems to be the number on the board, and each patient has four beeping machines on varied medication schedules, the game of "Beat the Clock" engulfs the nurse's entire shift.

I walk over to the station and try to be friendly. "It looks like today might be a little easier. There seem to be fewer patients on the floor than the day Gary was admitted."

A middle-aged nurse with kind eyes looks up and says, "Well, they didn't call in Suzy today, so it's really the same for us." Then it occurs to me, the hospital ramps up or down staff to meet demand.

I continue walking the floor and I see a mom pushing her son in a wheelchair. I've seen her before. Her son is in the room next to Gary. They're my new neighbors. This is the first time I've seen her child out of the room. I notice his head tilts way too much to his right side. He doesn't seem to be able to hold it up and his hands seem to flail randomly. He is adorable with big dark eyes. His physique seems normal. Something just recently must have happened, I guess. An accident? A brain injury? As the mother turns left, I glance at her face and notice she seems to have the weight of the world on her shoulders. My heart sinks, because unlike with Gary, I don't think an operation alone will help her child. I feel terrible for them. I turn right. I don't know what I'd say to her. As I walk down the hall, I notice what must be the boy's grandma in the lounge. She appears to be in her 70's and she's dressed in a lush, red sari. She is sitting with three other people. I decide to face my fear of not knowing what to say and choose to be neighborly.

"Hello." I figure it's a good start.

A younger male, 30-ish with the same complexion as the boy and his mom, quickly responds, "Hi. I've seen you here. How is your son?"

What a perfect thing to say. Here I am afraid to say the wrong thing. It's awkward for me to meet new people in this place. But he's right: Just show compassion. I can tell he is sincere in wanting to know. It is the opposite of what I experienced in corporate America, where the refrain is typically *It's not personal, it's business.*

"Thanks for asking, he is fine, just waiting for surgery. Who are you here for?" I ask, watching my behavior change in real time.

The man fumbles his tissue in his hand. He paces as he answers, "My nephew," he says. "He was hit by his school bus. He can't walk or talk, yet. It's a brain injury…"

Oh my God. What an awful thing to happen to a child and a family. A woman, who I assume is the boy's aunt, and looks like she's been crying, interrupts. "It's too soon to know the prognosis."

The boy's mom must have wheeled him around the entire floor and now wheels him into the lounge. As he enters, the family waves crazily with huge smiles on all of their faces, like they see him on the soccer field and want him to know they are in the stands. I notice a small smile on the boy's face. I'm trying not to focus on the spastic movements of his limbs. My heart is breaking for this family. To me the child looks like he'll never recover. But just as I am overwhelmed with sadness, the family seems delighted by his small gesture of happiness. They applaud, like his small smile scored the winning goal. I watch as his mom throws her arms around him and gives him a kiss.

I stand next to the wall quietly as the relatives whisper to each other. I don't know what they are saying, but their demeanor changes. The anxiety from before the smile vanishes. Describing what they look like is like trying to explain with words what a color looks like. I can't do it. But once you've seen it, you can recognize it over and over again. What I see on their faces is the look of love. If it were a color it would be the most beautiful color ever. As I leave the lounge I see this color shining deeper between families here more than any other place I've ever been.

How on earth can I analyze this from an operational point of view when this place clearly transcends a business perspective? At work, emotions are checked at the door. High-performing teams focus on issues. Maybe that's how hospital employees cope, too. But this place is clearly different.

I make my way back to Gary's room, walk in and stare at him sitting on the bed, hooked up to the beeping machines and laughing at a program on TV. I wrap my arms around him and kiss his forehead, just like the other mom. My son rolls his eyes. I hear three knocks on the door. Immediately, I think it is Dr. Stark, but instead it is a young woman in her 20's. She introduces herself as a child-life therapist. She explains that her role is to help families cope with hospitalizations. Her timing is perfect. I'm not a child but I need to talk. I can't process this place. She suggests we take a walk to the lounge.

Gary says, "See you guys later." We are interrupting his show.

We arrive in the well-worn lounge, with tissue boxes on side tables. The other family is gone. The therapist sits a little too close to me on the couch. In business meetings, I am used to more personal space. Her close proximity combined with missing Steve combined with my compromised emotional state compel me to confide in her. I start by giving the facts about Gary's condition in a business tone. But, sitting in the same chair as the other boy's grandma, unexpectedly overwhelms me. I feel so sad. Suddenly, I sob uncontrollably. I don't know what I am saying, but I ramble about the heartache of families. I say something about hope. I say something about love. I grab a tissue. I continue rambling and say, "Why Gary?"

All I know is she listens. She looks in my eyes, nodding. Eventually, she takes my hand. "You'll be OK. He'll be OK. I am here for you," she says in a soothing tone. She says nothing else. We just sit for what feels like forever. She even hugs me. Then, she walks me back to the room.

Once inside, I go to the desk and grab the "performance tracker." I ask her to write her name down on the list. She sees Marta Bazin starred. But she does not ask me why. She prints very legibly. Then she hands it directly to me.

"Thanks," I say. "I've decided to send a thank you letter to the CEO of the hospital recognizing the wonderful people who help us here." I place a huge star next to her name, place the paper back on the desk and I go and sit on the couch. She goes to Gary.

"I bet you wish you were home," she starts.

"Yeah." He is back to monosyllabic speech.

"What do you miss the most," she asks.

"Oh, my friends," Gary says. It is a couple more syllables. It's a start of him opening up, I think.

"What's going on back home?"

"Oh, they are trying to raise money for a water pump in Africa and they need my help," he says, as if all kids are concerned about getting clean water to a South African community.

"Really! That's cool. Have you ever been to South Africa?" she says. How did she know that this was the golden question to get him talking? He did so much press when he won the National Geographic trip. I hope he'll go into interviewee mode and not shut up.

"Oh yeah," Gary says, "National Geographic Kids took 15 winners with Lester Holt from NBC's 'Today' show. I went shark diving with the great whites. I saw lions mating, elephants fighting and leopards protecting their food in a tree." He says this in a sound bite, like it's the show opening.

"That's amazing. Did you meet the people?" She pulls up a chair next to his bed.

He speaks very deliberately and looks directly in her eyes. "It changed my life."

I interrupt. I want to give her some back story. (Since my outburst, I feel close to her. I typically don't cry my eyes out the first time I meet someone.) "Gary got to take me on the trip as well. I'd never been there either. But what I discovered is National Geographic Kids' mission is bigger than a fun trip to amazing places. National Geographic is more than experiencing great geography; it's about bringing closeness between cultures."

She ignores me. As she should.

"So, what were they like?" She asks the question directly to Gary. I get up from the couch and get a drink of water.

Gary answers, "I figured they were like us minus our technology, because before we went, National Geographic Kids had the winners raise money for a computer for their school." He presses the button to raise his bed so he can sit up better. She moves his tray out of the way as the head of the bed slowly rises. Gary continues, "Before we met the people, my mom and I had our own house to stay in! It was on the tip of South Africa overlooking the ocean. I stayed up late reading in the Jacuzzi. I thought people in South Africa lived like we do."

I interject again. I tell her it was beautiful, a horticulturist's paradise with exotic flowers and even a nursery on the property. I tell her our deck overlooked a wilderness expanse and that we had to stay inside at night because wild animals roamed. It was like something out of a movie. I know I'm behaving like my mom again, trying to take over the conversation, but I can't help myself.

"My mom's right," Gary says. "The whole thing seemed like a movie. Actually, National Geographic Kids and the 'Today' show kept filming us and getting our impressions. Like the time the lions were mating. I told my friend to say, 'You don't see that in a zoo!' They used it over and over again on TV."

"Wow, you saw a lot," the therapist says.

"Yeah, they do it every 15 minutes!"

Gary tells her that the townships left the greatest impression on him, lion mating notwithstanding.

"I remember the day our luxury bus pulled into the school. The girls and boys were there to greet us. The girls were dressed in straw skirts and the boys wore tribal shorts. They stood in two lines and raised their arms as we walked underneath them. They sang songs and danced when we entered their schoolyard. They looked so happy to see us. I made sure not to stare at the girls."

"Why?"

"Like I said, they wore straw skirts." He pauses, like he is painting a picture. She just looks at him quizzically.

I interject this time – appropriately – because I know he's embarrassed. "It's National Geographic – They were topless!"

Gary sighs. "We went into their school and it was empty. I mean no desks, no chairs, no books. The blackboard was so used and worn out in places you couldn't write anything. The kids do math with sticks in the sand outside."

"Wow." She adjusts her chair.

"But they seemed so much more joyful than the kids here, I mean not the kids here in the hospital. I mean the kids at my school. It was amazing. I played soccer with them. They had no grass, just a field of dirt. Most of them didn't have sneakers. The whole town came for the game. I still can hear them singing the songs on the sidelines. Know who won?"

"Who?"

"They beat us. We had sneakers, but they had spirit!"

The therapist asks Gary if he visited their homes and he tells her that the visits changed his life.

"Mom, you tell her. I need some water."

So I continue the story. I tell her about the township. How we saw home after home, thousands of people cramped together. Actually, they really are not homes; they are more like garden sheds made of paper and scraps of metal all right next to each other. There are no windows, just cut outs. I describe how I crossed from one "street" to another and I asked a local what the cord on the ground was and how he informed me it was a power line to tap into for electricity. Then he warned me to be careful because it was high voltage.

"I bet you were scared," she says. She is excellent at reflecting my feelings. I know this technique and it really works. It's the opposite of the power technique. It makes a person open up more because they feel you really understand them.

And that's what I do. I tell her about a young man who was standing outside his door. His home was maybe 120 square feet. Six people lived inside and they cooked on the grill outside. They shared the bathroom down the street with about 100 other people. They fetched water every day by walking about four miles round trip. The man worked seven days a week as a groundskeeper in the local tourist local lodge. Every year he got four weeks off to return home to his village to see his two daughters.

"I bet you were shocked." She pauses and says, "I mean not literally." All three of us burst out with a needed laugh.

One of the monitors beeps and a nurse comes in. There is so much more to the story but I notice for the first time that the therapist looks at her watch. Gary will have plenty of time to tell her how he's already sent over enough school supplies to fill two schools.

She gets up to leave and Gary announces, "Now, I am working to get them water. One water pump can supply 2,600 people."

"You're kidding me?" the therapist says as she opens the door.

"Nope. Since I'm here, I'm trying to coordinate with my friends on Facebook. We need to raise $14,000."

"You are incredible, Gary," she says. "I am sure you'll do it. You'll be out of here before you know it. Can I tell people in the hospital your story? We are always looking for special children and I think you are an inspiration."

"Sure." His monosyllable reminds me he is not interested in self-promotion. He really wants to just raise the money and send the people the water pump already.

"Thanks. I'll come back tomorrow to check in."

"Great."

The next three days move along, without incident. More and more people ask Gary to tell the story of South Africa. Someone even gives him $20 for the water pump!

He is no longer just another patient. We are building relationships. Gary is getting wonderful care and I have the list to prove it. We are making our new neighborhood part of our community.

What You Can Do Now

---

1. Decorate the room.

Ask loved ones to send cards, flowers, balloons ... anything cheerful. A cheery room really does help the patient feel they are part of a bigger community and they are remembered and cared about. People want to help and will ask what they can do. Let them help.

2. Create a high-performing team.

People love acknowledgement for a job well done. There are many new faces and I found it hard to keep them straight. Have each employee write down their name and job function. When they are done, acknowledge their effort. Commit to writing a "Thank you" letter to the CEO of the hospital when you leave. Write down what you thought of the interaction. I only let people who made a positive impact put their name on the list. Keep the list someplace visible. I found everyone wanted to be on the list.

3. Talk. Don't hold in your fear.

Find the hospital's family therapist, a friend, clergy or a relative. Anyone with some detachment from the immediate situation. They will have perspective and capacity to support you and listen. Let someone comfort you.

* * *

Chapter 7
Waiting for Emergency Surgery

My first night's sleep in the hospital is an oxymoron. Even if I do nod off, the monitors beeping and the ambulance sirens screaming remind me exactly where I am. My butt keeps slipping between two of the three cushions on the sofa. At least the nurses tend to be quiet through the night, checking on Gary every four hours.

Before dawn, the door flies open, the lights flash on and without my contacts in my eyes I can't make out more than fuzzy shapes hurrying toward Gary's bed. With my poor eyesight they could be aliens, but I think they are humans pressing on his belly. There are three of them, maybe four. They don't introduce themselves, even though they went right by me and this is the first morning I'm here. They are not nurses. Their gait is so much faster. I hear some talking and Gary just yelped. They must be the residents because they are so perky, like it is the middle of the day. I've heard they start rounds super early. Gary is just as perky. "Know what today is?" he bursts out after one resident finishes pressing on his stomach.

"October 26th," a resident pronounces, like it's an easy answer on a test.

"Oh maybe, I don't know," Gary says. "I've been here too long. No, today is the day. It's my surgery day." Gary's enthusiasm shines brighter to me than the florescent lights that I am now squinting from as I try to compose myself.

"Yes. Let me push on your belly again," a different resident requests. He writes down data and does not acknowledge Gary's big day. Another resident asks Gary about his pain level. A five. He records the number. This seems to be the same information the nurses took when they checked earlier.

I say hello. They say hello back but I don't know if they're looking at me. They get back to collecting data. I wonder if the residents think of Gary by his name or his medical condition. He's probably the teenage boy with Crohn's awaiting surgery. Maybe their description to their superiors adds in more medical terminology, but no first name. After my tears yesterday, I sort of grasp the need for lack of emotional attachment to the patient, but I don't like it. Especially when it's my son they are dealing with.

I will not get off the couch because I am sleeping in one of Steve's XXL T-shirts and my undies. Another reason is that my hair looks like I've been electrocuted. It always does after a night's sleep. My hair is curly and long and it frizzes up when I toss and turn on the pillow. My kids are embarrassed by the bride-of-Frankenstein look I achieve effortlessly every morning. Occasionally, I'll threaten, "If you don't do this, I'll go to your classroom with my morning hair." It is scary enough for them to conform. Gary doesn't say it, but I know he's happy I'm basically hiding under the blanket.

All of a sudden, the lights go dark and the residents exit at the same speed of their entry. They say nothing to me about Gary's progress or anything about what they observe. A couple of minutes later, a nurse comes quietly to remind Gary, "No food today. It's surgery day." She only turns on some under-lighting so as not to jar him from rest. But he is too excited and doesn't seem to notice her thoughtfulness.

"It's my big day," Gary exclaims to the nurse.

"I know. Just remember, don't eat. They can't operate if you eat," she repeats.

Gary looks over at me and tells me, "Go downstairs and grab yourself some breakfast. But please bring it back, just in case the doctors stop by. I want you here. It's my big day, Mom."

"I know. I'll be quick," I say. I head into the shower to wash my frizzy hair. After drying myself off, I put some gel in my palm and spread it over my wet head, so my hair will dry with long ringlets. I choose to look professional today. I am in a place of business – to me, the most important business – ensuring my son's health. Instead of sweats or jeans I wear business casual attire. I imagine I am going to have lots of meetings today. I dress in the bathroom and check that my hair looks respectable in the mirror. I am not used to sharing a room with Gary. I open the bathroom door and Gary says, "You look great, Mom, now hurry!"

I run down to the cafeteria for a bagel. As instructed, I bring it back to the room but this time I feel bad. As usual Gary is hooked up to the beeping machines, but his bedside tray is empty. No breakfast served. I feel guilty eating in front of him. I break off bird-size bites and turn my head as I put them in my mouth. He must sense my angst. He says, "I can't eat, Mom. But you need to be strong. So eat!" I nibble three bites for basic sustenance. I double-check to see his reaction. He seems fine. I am hungry and I don't want to become weak so I nibble a little more. He's right, this is a big day. I need to be strong.

Still, I don't finish the whole thing and just as I chuck out the rest in the trash, Steve enters the room. It's not even 8 a.m. and he is already here. I throw my arms around him and give him a big kiss. Steve's presence fills me with love. "Today is your day!" Steve says, running over to Gary. I'm not surprised that Steve knows exactly what to say to his son. One of the reasons I married Steve is that he is in tune with other people's feelings, no matter what he is going through.

There is no schedule of events for the day. We are told they will come and get Gary when it is time. We just need to wait. As the morning drags on, Gary gets out of bed and moves his multi-pump hook-up so he can sit on the couch next to his dad. On Steve's lap is my laptop. Steve drapes his arm over Gary's shoulder and they watch "The Three Stooges." Gary is cracking up at the slapstick and Steve's laughter is so loud, I finally have something to drown out the beeping machines. I look around the room and take a mental picture. I capture my men laughing as if they don't have a care in the world. In the background of this picture is a wall full of bright colorful balloons and cute stuffed animals. If the balloons didn't say "Get Well," the cheerful display would look like a birthday party. In this moment love overpowers our distressing situation. I actually feel happy sitting in a hospital room awaiting a complex surgery that involves removing an undisclosed amount of my son's intestines. Another oxymoron.

They laugh and laugh the morning away. The one-moment snapshots are Steve's gift to me. Steve is a pro at building wonderful moment memories. I learned from him how to take each moment and live it now, not worry about the next moment. I've learned I cannot deprive myself of this moment because my next moment might be worse.

By afternoon Gary and Steve have progressed (maybe digressed) to watching Bugs Bunny as a concert pianist who shoots an audience member for coughing too much. They burst out in laughter. Nurses come in periodically to check on medication levels and we just wait. Gary takes a break from the laughter to go to the bathroom. I hear him screaming the "F" bomb from the bathroom but this time he adds, "It will be over today. I can make it." Then he adds another "F" bomb but it's long and drawn out. Like it's the last time he'll need to say it, so he maximizes the duration. As the word sounds in the background, the phone rings. It's Dr. Simmon calling. His "hello" sounds tentative and I figure something is up. We have not seen him all day or heard from the surgeon.

"Randi, we need to move Gary's surgery out one day. There is an emergency surgery and it will be too late for Dr. Carroll to start Gary's surgery today. I hope you understand."

What else can I say but, "Sure." Dr. Simmon thanks me and hangs up.

Simultaneously, the bathroom door opens up. Even though I know Gary is in pain because he always is after urinating, his smiling face appears. I know he will be devastated with this news. I can't imagine holding my emotions together if I were hungry and waiting so long and then told to wait another whole day. I'd lose it.

I've seen so many kids lose it in the hospital. It's a place for disappointment and pain. I see many parents try their best to console their children with lots of tissues, kisses and hugs. When I eavesdrop, I hear them apologizing, as if it's their fault. I bet a lot of life-long emotional family baggage happens from a hospital stay. The children get obstinate. Many times I hear the parents use the bribing technique. The kids learn how to get what they want. It is a vicious cycle. The doctors deal with the physical symptoms but getting a kid to "like" getting shots or giving blood or drinking barium is the parent's job.

I think Gary needs to feel less like a victim of circumstance and more like he's in control. The feeling of power is something I can give him using some of my management motivational techniques. If he needs a tissue and a hug, I can offer these up as well.

So, I take a deep breath and instead of telling him the news, I try to get his buy-in on postponing the surgery by giving him the choice. I learned in GE, if an employee has a choice he or she will move to action in a more positive way, even if the choice is the lesser of two evils. So, like a manager and not a mother, I say, "Gary, the doctor called and he had an emergency surgery today. We've been waiting all day for your surgery to begin, but it looks like he can't start till tonight and he'll be tired. He can start early tomorrow morning, rested. Which is better for you?" I feel like I hoodwinked him, but I know it will help him accept the circumstances.

"I want him rested, Mom," he says.

"That's what he wants too. Can you hang in till Tuesday?" I say, hoping the answer is obvious.

"Sure, Mom." He gets the answer right but his smile fades as he moves the pumping machine toward his bed. With each step, I see the pain return. It's late afternoon. I figure he must be starved. I hit the "concierge button" and Laura, the experienced nurse, comes by.

"Can he eat if the surgery won't be till tomorrow?" I ask, hoping for a little reprieve for Gary.

"No, he needs to have an empty belly," she says firmly. I can tell there are no exceptions to this rule. Thank goodness Gary understands the word "No." Starting when Gary was a toddler, I never changed my mind after I delivered the "no" word. I knew he wouldn't try to finagle an exception to this rule either.

"It's OK, Mom. I'll wait it out. It will be better if Dr. Carroll is rested. I've waited this long. It's one more day."

"That's my boy," Steve exclaims. "You get it!"

Laura looks at Gary and says, "You do get it. This is just a blip. You'll be fine."

I like that Laura is treating Gary as a person. I like that she is helping to give him perspective. Maybe she is right. We need to look at this as a blip. No one's life is a straight line.

I walk over to Gary and give him a high-five. Steve tells me to go downstairs and grab some dinner. He'll stay with Gary until I return and then he'll go home to Matt and Grandma. I know he lost a work day but neither of us says anything and no one asks. Steve is managing three ambulatory surgery facilities now, and the pressure is intense.

My second night in the hospital, I place a sheet over the three cushions and tuck it tightly. I am hoping to prevent my tushy slipping through the cracks again. Gary and I watch TV until we fall asleep. I must have slept through the night without the nurses waking me because I am awakened from a sound sleep by the large door bursting open and the overhead lights flashing on. My alarm clock. The fuzzy figures of three residents stand over Gary. Unlike yesterday, his yelps sound groggy. He must have been sleeping too. The fuzzy figures talk loudly as if they've been up for hours and we all should be up too. Again, they ask the same questions as the nurses. They must have access to the same data as the nurses but from what I can tell, they don't ask the nurses for their information.

I figure somehow waking up the patient must be protocol, because they do it every day to every patient without apologizing. It's like the patient is a piece of equipment. You do not need to talk to widgets; you can just test them, capture data and try to find a way to fix the machinery. It is the same approach I feel they take with my son. I've seen different residents all week and never really talk with them about Gary. They seem very busy. They come across like they are collecting data for a research project and they want an "A." However, my guess is the grade does not include a patient relations portion. They seem to just care about getting Gary's engine to run properly, in this case his intestines.

After the residents leave, I shower, put the gel in my hair, and dress in slacks with a cable knit sweater. I go down for my breakfast. I carefully choose to eat oatmeal and avoid the gooey sticky cinnamon bun that seems to call out to me. The frosting is melting over the top and the smell is scrumptious. But, I know food cannot comfort me. I am not going down that path. A young resident stands in the checkout line behind me. The resident wears his crisp white coat with shiny stethoscope hanging over his neck with pride. He looks like one of the residents that touched Gary's belly the last two mornings, but I'm not sure because of the contacts. Maybe he recognizes my hair. I look directly at him, waiting to see if he'll say hello. He looks down at his tray. I pay and wait for him at the utensil station. As he reaches for a fork, I smile to see if he'll acknowledge me.

Nothing.

"Good morning," I start off.

"Good morning," he says and walks off with the other resident, who also looks familiar, and who also says nothing to me.

I head back to the elevator and Dr. Stark is coming right toward me. I look directly at her and she looks at me and then looks down at the ground. I know she recognizes me! I feel sick inside. These people are "caring" for my son but they don't acknowledge me. I realize the mission here is to fix the patient. Nothing else matters and maybe it shouldn't. Maybe I am expecting too much. Politeness is a courtesy, though not a measured protocol.

Today is supposedly the big day, but after yesterday, I think we've learned that anything can happen. Gary is clearly not as perky as yesterday. He is hungry. The lack of food has drained his energy. In the room a trio of doctors visit at different times. I've never met two of them. The doctors explain what they're going to do. They want us to sign forms. I glance down at one of the forms and see "A risk of death." Once I see that, I just want the surgery to be finished already. I'm not hearing them. It's all a blur. There are a lot of words on the document and I've been trained to read everything I sign. I ask for a couple of minutes to review the documents. The doctors hand them to me and leave. Between phone calls of friends and relatives wishing Gary well, the forms lay on the desk, unsigned. The nurse comes in to remind me to sign the document. It is clearly a legal document written by lawyers to protect the hospital but I am not represented with counsel. The only choice I have is to be slow to sign and try to understand the real risks associated with the surgery. For the first time on this trip, it seems the clock is ticking.

The morning progresses and Steve returns, looking like he hasn't slept. Matt and Grandma are faring well, he says, and are thinking of Gary. As Steve takes out the laptop to watch "I Love Lucy" reruns with Gary, the nurse reminds us to sign the form. Steve reviews the consent form and says it's pretty standard. I try to absorb the document, but can't. I tell her to come back. As the day ticks along she comes back two more times with the reminder. They are ready to begin surgery but won't until the forms are signed. I bet almost 100 percent of the parents just sign the first time. Even with my holdout, Steve comforts me and says it's protocol, we have to sign. He takes a pen and signs because finally time is critical. Within minutes of our signature, an attendant comes to wheel Gary's stretcher to surgery. I walk in the bright halls next to Gary's stretcher, holding back tears. I feel my heart pounding. I wouldn't be surprised if the attendant could see my sweater move with the beat of my heart. As the elevator drops from the sixth floor to the third floor, I feel like I am in a slow motion dream and I can't wake up. And I can't scream. I realize this is a time of faith. I am so glad I believe in God because I'm terrified. I just pray.

In the admitting O.R. area, everyone announces their names and their roles. Apparently they've had training in patient relations.

"Hi, I'm Nancy. I will take your child to the operating room."

"Hi, I'm Sally. I will be the nurse during the operation."

"Hi, I'm Dr. Klein. I will be the anesthesiologist."

I just smile at them. How many people are on this team? I don't know and can't find a way to care about them. I look down at Gary. He is calm and appears ready for surgery. It's his last hope to get rid of this pain and I presume he is not concerned about any of the risks.

"Hi, I'm Audrey. I am the recovery room nurse. You can wait up in your son's room. We will call you there when he is in recovery. It should be about four hours."

I stand with Steve next to Gary's gurney and think about "moment memories." I decide to follow Steve's lead and live in the moment. I need Gary to feel good about this whole experience. I suspect he feels bad that our family life is disrupted by his illness. He's not stupid. He knows the sacrifice his brother, Grandma and even the dog are making by having his parents in the hospital. I don't want him to feel bad. But how do I convince him that spending a week in a hospital is a positive experience for a parent?

I try to imagine a positive experience, one completely opposite from my experience here so far. I've never been to a spa, but I've seen magazine articles where all you do is eat veggies, exercise and have massages and facials. I could do that sort of thing here with all this time on my hands. I tell Gary my plans as he waits to be rolled in. "Gary, guess what? During your recovery, I'm going to get healthier too. While you're here I'm going to be with you every step of the way. And this will give me some 'me' time! I never get that. I am going to treat this place like my personal health spa."

"You're crazy, Mom. It's a hospital, not a spa," he says.

"Yes, I know. But now I can have my food prepared for me, I can read all day, I can bathe all night and I can even go on the massage chair whenever I want. I am going to exercise every day and take power walks on the floor. By the time you get out of here, we'll both feel great!"

"Mom, I'm gonna make sure you do 25 push-ups every day. See you later."

And with that statement, they take my son.

Steve takes my hand. We watch them roll Gary to the back of the room until he disappears. We walk into the hall and look at each other. I think he gives me a hug. I feel numb.

"He'll be better soon," Steve says, with hope in his voice. "They will cut out the diseased intestine and fix his bladder." I guess that's what they're going to do; it's the right thing to say.

With four hours to wait, Steve suggests we grab some lunch from the cafeteria. This time I take the time to look around. I'm supposed to be starting my spa. The room is painted for kids, in a galaxy theme. I look up to the ceiling and notice a skylight through which I can see big puffy clouds. The world outside is moving forward but we're not going anywhere. I am not hungry but I know I need to stay strong. So I grab a water and salad. I really want to throw up. Steve and I sit at a table for two and eat our lunch. Silently. This is so unlike us. We seem to be just like a lot of parents in the cafeteria, though. Perhaps they are waiting for a surgery to be over as well. To me, waiting is the worst part. I have no control. I hope those people I saw on the surgery floor are competent. I have no idea how long they have been working here. Are they newbies? Are they typically on the same team? Or do they have a learning curve because they are not familiar with each other? I like to know these things. It gives me comfort. Even if everything goes perfectly, I fear that Gary will have a long recovery ahead. I hope Gary goes to sleep smiling at the idea of us growing stronger together here.

Steve and I toss our half-eaten lunches in the trash can. We go back up to the room to wait. We sit on the couch and wait. Steve's eyes slowly close. His long legs jut out on the floor and his head falls back against the wooden couch frame. He's going to sleep away the wait. I can't. My mind races. I open my laptop to check out the news and read about the world's problems. I visit MSNBC's website. There is an article about health insurance costs. This article's timing coincides with President Obama's push for health care reform. It's been in the news a lot lately. The health bill is 2,700 pages long. Every day, newspaper articles describe how our Congressmen and Senators do not have time to read the bill. But, with a majority of Democrats in control, the Health Reform Act is expected to pass. One of the main provisions in the bill is to eliminate the ability of health care insurance companies to deny coverage for pre-existing conditions. It's causing an uproar because many people think it will drive up costs. To me, I am so grateful because Gary may be uninsurable without it. What else is happening with the reform? With Steve sleeping, I click the link and peruse the article. It's an exposé on health insurance costs and families being financially wiped out. Of all days, today is the day I read this! I don't want to think about the cost of care. Not now. I just want the surgery to be over! The story has video links too. I can't deny that I have to deal with my reality. So, I click the first video.

I see a middle-aged couple, with graying hair, just like Steve and me. They are sitting in a living room. The wife tells how hospital expenses wiped out their family savings. They had to move. Their child eventually died. They look like they've been hit by a train. I start to cry. I pray to God that Gary is doing OK. I look at Steve and he is still asleep.

I click the next video. The father lost his job and his insurance. They racked up $100,000 of medical bills.

I click the next story. This family has coverage but it turns out there is a cap on their coverage. Their child has a chronic disease and hit the cap by the age of 18. I look at the background of where they are being interviewed. It's a one-bedroom crummy apartment. They look exhausted and defeated. Yet I have a hunch that at one time they seemed just like us.

As I click from one family's story to the next, I realize that they all ended up with the same devastating financial outcomes. A new sense of panic enters my body. Before this surgery, not one person mentioned anything about the cost or our insurance deductible, or limits on our coverage or anything. We didn't think about it either. I have no idea how much money the doctors are charging or what the daily hospital room rate is. It seems to me as if cost is no object. I appreciate that this is the system; there is no way I could make a financial trade-off over Gary's health. With my child under the knife, I totally understand cost shouldn't be an issue. I just want him better. But it's an ideological world that I just realized might collapse once the bills come in. With Steve's new job at half his previous pay, I understand financial instability. I shake Steve. He does not respond. I shake him again before he opens his eyes.

"Honey, are we covered for this?" I say.

"Sure we are," he says groggily. I am not sure he knows what I am talking about.

"Really? Our insurance covers the cost? How do you know?" I say but don't wait for his response. Trying to respect that he did just wake up, I whisper, "This other family found out afterwards they were not covered." I realize I'm too frantic to care about his sleep and blurt out loud, "How much does this cost?"

"I don't know!" he says, now awake. He looks at me. "We are covered. We must be."

I continue reading and watching. The article explains how medical bills can run into hundreds of thousands of dollars. It explains how no one tells you about any costs. Or compares options based on costs. They just keep trying something to get you better and that's a good thing, isn't it? The article talks about all the testing, which runs up costs and increases revenue for the hospital. The article concludes that you need to know what your plan covers.

Except for our little white plastic insurance card tucked in my wallet, I've never read anything about the written plan. I have no idea what our deductible is, if there is a cap and if this doctor is covered. I can't remember anyone in the hospital reviewing our insurance coverage with us. They did make sure we *had* coverage, though. It was the first thing they asked for in the emergency room. So, they know they are covered. How can I even be thinking about this while Gary is in surgery?

"Steve, call your human resources department now!" I am hysterical.

I hand Steve the cellphone. Steve calls his human resources department. They are in California. Someone on the other end says to him they will get back to him tomorrow. Now, I worry about the outcome of Gary's surgery *and* the hospital bill.

Steve closes his eyes. I do Sudoku puzzles over and over again. I've done so many that even the hard ones only take me 15 minutes. Three hours later my phone rings. "He's fine," someone says. "Come down and see him in recovery." I jump up and open the door and shout out to Steve, "He's fine. Let's go!"

I want to race down to see Gary, but the elevator stops on four on the way down. An orderly enters and smiles widely with a missing tooth and a smell of cigarettes so strong, I gag. I cover my nose as the worker stares at me and I push the third floor button repeatedly. Let me out. Let me out of the elevator. The third floor button is lit and I still push it relentlessly. Almost in rhythm I say to myself, *Let me out of this hospital.*

We step out of the elevator and Steve grabs my hand and pulls me back as I try to race to the recovery room. I know he is trying to calm me down. I yank my hand away in a tiff and walk faster. I look at my watch. It's 6 p.m. There are no windows in the hallway and, despite all the lights, the area seems dark. Everything feels dark.

I burst through the double doors to the recovery room and the nurse points to the back stall. Gary seems to be resting comfortably. He is hooked up to a new pumping machine. I just stare at him and reach for Steve's hand. As I watch Gary's breaths, I realize this is the same stall he was in after his colonoscopy, three years earlier. I eerily remember the layout of the floor. There's the bathroom, right where I remember. I flash back to the first time I was in this stall when the doctor stood right where I am now and said, "Gary, you have Crohn's disease." Standing in the same place, I am flooded with memories of how Gary, Steve and I got to this place to begin with.

Three years ago, Gary was 12 years old, weighed only 83 pounds and was 4 feet 10 inches tall. He dashed to the bathroom after every meal. Steve and I feared he might have an eating disorder. He'd push the food around on his plate and barely eat. What we didn't know was that he had constant diarrhea and needed to use the bathroom 20 times a day. Gary never complained of pain. He was very active and a good student. Every season he played a sport. In fall there was football; in winter there was basketball; and in the spring, tennis. At his birthday party, at his favorite restaurant, I noticed Gary was looking and behaving differently than the other kids. Gary used to be bigger than they were but now he was shorter and skinny. At the party the other boys ate and ate just like I heard boys do. But, not Gary. He ate food, but he didn't scarf it down like his friends did.

So, I started to pay attention more when he was around other boys. That winter when I took him to basketball games, he didn't run down the court at full blast. He looked exhausted and after the game, even if the team won, he'd shy away from the other boys. He barely talked. But he told me he didn't want to quit the team. Yet, he seemed frustrated with the boys not passing the ball to him. I explained the basics to him, like the kids aren't going to pass you the ball if you don't run and try to create a shot. The coach is not going to give you play time if you don't play hard. You'll have to practice your free throws. It seemed so obvious to me. He'd listen but didn't ever practice. Because he said he wanted to play, I wanted to support him. I turned into a barking drill sergeant mom. "Did you practice your free throws today?" or "C'mon let's go outside and shoot some hoops." But he always claimed he was too tired. Without any symptoms of pain, and except for sleeping a lot, like I'd been told most teenagers do, I did not take him to the doctor. I don't think I was in denial. I had no idea something was physically wrong. I thought he was lazy. Despite the fact that Gary would always say he wanted to improve on the field or in the classroom, his actions did not reflect his words.

I knew my barking drill sergeant mothering technique was wrong. I hated doing it. "Brush your teeth. Remember your coat. Did you put the math homework in your backpack?" From all my management experience, I knew motivation must come from within. Micromanagers fail at creating self-starters because employees learn to just wait for the commands. When I worked for one, I worked in fear because my micromanager constantly yelled at me, just like I was doing to Gary. I recognized this. I looked for another technique. Luckily for Gary, despite all of my mom's crazy ways, she'd taught me what her grandma from the *shtetl* in Russia had taught her: "You have to work with what you have." I bet that is how they found happiness with so little. I decided to quit the barking drill sergeant mom technique cold turkey.

After a basketball game where Gary played terribly and his team lost, instead of barking at him for his lackadaisical performance on the court, I asked him how he was feeling when we came home. He sat on his bed grasping a brown worn-out teddy bear on his lap. He couldn't find words to express himself. He seemed so lost. He started to tear up. But he didn't say anything. My heart broke. I didn't know why but the world seemed to be whizzing by him. He seemed so confused. I realized Gary needed help to get through every day. "Honey," I said, "I have a secret list that can help you. If you follow the list you can learn to do anything."

He looked up at me. I think he expected the drill sergeant mom to appear and seemed relieved. He let go of the bear. He went to his desk and tore off a piece of paper from a notebook. He came back to the bed and handed me a pen.

I wrote down a list of five things he needed to do every day:

1. **Eat right**
2. **Get enough sleep**
3. **Exercise**
4. **Finish your to-do list**
5. **Never lie to yourself**

He got up from the bed and put the list on his desk. I watched him over the next few weeks try to eat more as well as complete the rest of the steps. One day as he was doing some homework, he called me into his room. He picked up the piece of paper and pointed to number five.

"Ah, the good ol' number five." I said it with humor because I knew whatever he was going to tell me was important.

"Mom, I'm too tired to finish my math and I have diarrhea all the time. That's why I go to the bathroom. My stomach hurts a lot." He looked like he'd shared the secret of the world and already felt some of the burden lifted. I felt awful.

"You've been pretending to be fine, Gary?" I said it softly.

"Uh huh." He'd never mentioned any pain before. I wish he'd told me sooner, but was so glad he was finally speaking up. I returned to the list.

"Gary, many grownups don't have the courage to be truly honest with themselves. You should be proud of yourself," I told him. "I'm so sorry you've had to go through this. I'll help you find a way to feel better." I wrapped my arms around him and squeezed.

The next day our journey started with an appointment to Gary's pediatrician to tell her about his pain and diarrhea. She followed protocol and made a referral to a gastroenterologist who followed protocol and prescribed an upper and lower G.I. The G.I. exam passed a camera through the intestines to see if anything was internally wrong, standard protocol for a Crohn's diagnosis. Well, after the G.I. exam, Gary ended up at this same stall the first time.

Now, I see a nurse finishing up some paperwork and I snap back to reality. Is the doctor coming? What feels like a long time was probably just a couple of minutes since we arrived by Gary's side. Steve and I just stare at the regular rhythm of Gary's breathing. He seems so calm. I grab Steve's hand. I actually take a "moment memory" picture, because Gary hasn't always been this calm in this hospital.

Three years ago, the first time Gary prepped for an X-ray of his intestines, he had to drink barium. This is a beginning step for an irritable bowel disorder diagnosis, like Crohn's or colitis. I do not wish any child to have to drink this stuff. According to Gary it is horrible. But according to the gastroenterologist it is critical. Barium must be drunk prior to a CT scan to allow for better computer tomography of the gastrointestinal tract. Patients have to fast prior to drinking the liquid which looks like a thin milkshake, sort of like liquid chalk. Even when it's flavored with chocolate, kids hate it. The barium sulfate gives the drink a mild acidic burning sensation. You're not allowed to chug it to get it out of the way; you have to pace the drinking of the potion. A patient typically begins 90 minutes to two hours prior to the CT scan. The nurses tell you how much to consume and when. Then, even when you think you are done, a small portion is reserved for just before the test. This ensures that as much of the gastrointestinal tract as possible is coated and the child is fully miserable.

No one told us this before the test. I never looked it up on Wikipedia. The nurse with a big smile asked Gary if he wanted the chocolate or strawberry flavor. Gary grinned and said "chocolate" like he was ordering ice cream. This was a cruel trick. He thought he was getting a chocolate shake but after one sip he declared, "I hate it. I am not drinking this stuff." The nurse looked over and informed me that he had to drink the whole thing in the next 90 minutes. Then, she walked out.

This was a nightmare. I couldn't drink it for him (unlike a middle school project, which the teacher knows the parents completed at the last minute when the kid couldn't get it together). Gary had to drink it. We were crowded under glaring florescent lights with other parents and children passing us to the X-ray room and I had to get Gary to drink the barium within a couple of hours. Then, we had to wait up to four hours for it to pass through his system. I was terrified that Gary would throw his first tantrum ever. He'd held it together his whole life, partly because I'd always been able to redirect him to avoid outbursts. Now, at 12 years old, it was just part of his nature to find alternatives. However, this time there seemed to be no other options.

Looking at him staring at the Styrofoam cup containing the barium, sitting in this busy hall, I realized I was the only other team member he had. The nurse certainly left. The doctor wasn't involved in this part of the process. He'd never even told us about this obstacle. It's the parents who are expected to get their child to drink the stuff. If anyone was going to get a kid to be the poster child for drinking barium it was me. I'm used to building high-performing teams at work, so I figured I could to use those same skills to motivate Gary. But unlike employees who often try to put their best face forward, Gary dug in.

"It's horrible. I won't drink it."

I counted to 10, in my head, and with each passing number encouraged the patience to flow in my blood stream. If I forced him, he'd rebel.

"Honey, I know it is horrible and I hate that you have to go through this," I told him. "But the doctors want to figure out what is wrong so you can get strong and grow. They have to see your insides. This drink will allow them to do that. Do you want to grow again?"

"Yep."

"Ah, then we have to get through *only* one hour so you can grow for years." I paused. I smiled. I waited for his response. The hardest part of motivating others is sometimes shutting up. I needed to sell Gary on drinking this stuff. In sales, I've learned if I am talking, I am not selling. I stayed silent until he spoke. It felt like an eternity.

"One hour?" he said.

"Uh huh. One hour. I know it's tough so let's take it one swig at a time." I started to break down the overwhelming task of drinking the whole cup into manageable pieces. "In 15 minutes you just need to drink to here." I pointed on the small cup. "¼" looked really small. Fifteen minutes seemed like a long time for such a small amount.

He took less than a swig, maybe a sip, and said, "It's awful. It tastes like shit."

Now, cursing was not what I wanted my kid to do, especially in the middle of a crowded hall with other parents and their little kids. But Gary seemed empowered to be a middle-schooler and cursing. I knew I could use that.

"OK, I get it. It tastes really bad."

Gary rolled his eyes. "Like shit, Mom." He repeated the curse loud. Clearly, my son has seen me use the reflection technique before in which I restated his feeling to show him I heard him. Now, he wanted me to acknowledge how bad it really was.

"OK, how about every time you drink a whole swig, you get to curse and I won't say a thing."

He tilted his head like in disbelief. "Really?" He sounded a little excited.

"Yep, go for it." I smiled and sat back in my chair.

Gary started to attack the eight ounces. He cursed quietly. I think he, too, didn't want the other little kids to hear him or maybe he didn't want to scare them. The nurses did not hear him cursing, but they did stop by periodically and notice his progress. A couple remarked how well he was progressing. At the 60-minute mark,

Gary slammed the cup down on the armrest. He turned it over. Not a drop came out. One nurse, a stocky woman who looked liked she'd been working in the department a very long time, saw the empty cup. She walked over to Gary and said, "I wish other kids could be so brave."

Gary smiled wide. He hadn't been able to perform as well as other kids for a long time. I did not know it at the time, but the diarrhea was robbing him of nutrition. His iron level was drastically low. It should have been around 50 milligrams but his was about 12. That's why he was always tired. After simply drinking eight ounces of barium, he felt good about his accomplishment. I was so grateful to that one nurse who took the time to acknowledge his progress. She made him feel special. I thanked her and I think she knew the importance of her pat on Gary's back. She made a big difference that day.

Steve squeezes my hand, bringing me back to the present. Gary looks like he is stirring. We call out to him but he doesn't respond. I look down the hall to see if the doctor is coming yet, but I don't see him. A nurse stops by and checks the monitors. She tells us it won't be long before the doctor checks in. The last time Gary was in this same stall, he woke up quickly. He did not have as much anesthesia that time. Waiting for the doctor also felt like an eternity. When the doctor arrived back then, Gary sat up quickly and tilted his head, the same way my dad tilted his head while waiting for his prognosis. Then Gary actually said, "What's up, Doc?" just like my dad had. I saw my father's strength inside Gary and felt my father's presence.

When the doctor unloaded the words: "Gary, you have Crohn's disease," I didn't know what Crohn's disease was. It didn't sound good and Dr. Simmon had a real serious look on his face. But seeing Gary looking at the doctor the same way my dad looked at his doctor, I knew Gary had my father's strength. I looked up to God and whispered, "Thank you."

Now, after today's surgery, Gary is literally in the same place as where he first received his diagnosis.

When I look down the hall I see the surgeon, Dr. Carroll, walking quickly toward the stall. He is thin like a runner and has an easygoing smile. This time there is too much anesthetic in Gary to wake up when Dr. Carroll comes in the room. The doctor looks at Gary and turns to us.

"He'll be fine," he says. "I took out the diseased intestine."

I ask exactly what he did in the operating room. The doctor looks around for a place for us to sit but there are not enough chairs. I bet he is tired from standing so long. He suggests going to the empty waiting room. Gary seems to be resting comfortably and a nurse is heading toward his stall. Steve and I follow the doctor to a dimly lit waiting room. The doctor sits down and we follow suit.

"What did you do?" I ask again.

He answers with a word that sounds like it has lots of letters and means nothing to me. I must look confused because he says, "Let me show you."

After a four-hour surgery, the doctor searches in his pocket for a piece of paper he can use to illustrate the surgery. He finds a crumpled piece of paper and flattens it out with his hands, then grabs a pen and starts drawing the intestinal tract. It's amazing to me that these doctors don't carry preprinted pads of the digestive tract to use to describe operations. As he draws a diagram, he announces, "This is the esophagus. This is the stomach. This is the large intestine and the small intestine." I look down at his diagram and he is clearly not an artist nor should he be. I can't tell one body part from the other.

"I removed two inches of small intestine and five inches of large intestine and reattached the ends. I took out Gary's appendix, ileum and cecum and re-sewed the hole in his bladder from the fistula of where the appendix secured itself. I did it laparoscopically. Gary has one main incision and three small holes." The doctor's calm voice makes it sound like this is not a big deal, but it sounds like a much bigger procedure than I'd expected.

I stare at the picture wondering what those things do that he took out. I only recognize the appendix, which no one had mentioned any plans to remove, including when they were having me sign waivers.

"I've put him on I.V. antibiotics so he doesn't get an infection," the doctor says. "The first 24 hours we need to watch his temperature. Gary will stay in recovery for about an hour and then we'll transfer him to his room. He'll not remember much the first two days. Do you have any questions?"

It's a polite thing to ask but he is already moving to stand up and I can see he wants to go. It is late. I do not know what to ask anyway. The doctor says Gary will be fine. I just have to trust that the surgeon did what he's supposed to do.

"Maybe tomorrow," I respond, leaving myself an opening for continuing the conversation.

"I'll stop by and see Gary in the morning," Dr. Carroll says as he gets up and walks out.

He did his job today. Everyone did their job today. He wants to go home. But I feel like I still don't understand the big picture. Is Gary going to be pain-free? Will he still be sick? Is this bad dream over?

Steve and I walk slowly to the recovery room. We stare at Gary sleeping, hooked up to the machines, with nurses coming in periodically to check on him. Steve moves Gary's cotton covering and looks at the bandages on his stomach. There seem to be four places the doctor cut open, three small and one pretty large. Steve wells up and I take his hand. A male attendant arrives to transfer Gary back to his room.

I wish we could all be together here tonight but Steve wants to go home to Matt. In addition, he has to work in New Jersey tomorrow and our home is much closer to his job. So Steve walks with me and Gary's gurney to the elevator. Steve pushes the down button to go home and the attendant pushes the up button to take Gary and me back to the sixth floor. The down elevator arrives first. Steve bends down and kisses Gary. He looks up at me and takes my hands. He doesn't need to say anything. I stand on my tippy toes to reach up to kiss him. Just then another elevator arrives. The attendant starts to move Gary inside. Steve gently waves his hand prodding me to go. The protocol train keeps moving.

We return to the room and I feel like I've been up all night, even though it's probably not past eight. I'm glad I don't see any clocks on the walls because seeing the time would make me even more tired. The sight of the night duty nurse waiting by Gary's room confirms that the shifts have already changed.

The night duty nurse is a man in his 30's, physically fit and self-assured. We haven't had a male nurse. He looks directly in my eyes as he tells me his name, Jeff. He looks down at Gary on the gurney and seems to do a quick assessment. He says Gary will be fine. Then Jeff says hello to the attendant. The friendly casualness of their exchange seems like they respect being males in a predominantly female workplace.

Jeff busily hooks up five bags of fluids to a pump that regulates the drips through Gary's I.V. It's the same kind of beeping machine they used before the surgery. The nurse moves swiftly and confidently, checking and rechecking the bags, reading prescription amounts and looking at the digital indicators. I don't know what all the fluids are for or how much Gary needs. I'm too tired to talk and ask questions. But the nurse seems to be particularly attentive. He seems to have lots of time and is not rushing. Gary is a couple of hours post–op and according to the doctor the first 48 hours are critical. Watching Jeff's attention to detail, I like him instantly and feel calmer with him in control.

I remove the three top cushions from the couch, place the white fitted sheet on the bottom cushions and find two blankets in the closet. I am so tired; I could sleep even if the crack of the cushions is the size of the Grand Canyon tonight. I go into the bathroom to change into Steve's XXL T-shirt and take out my contact lenses and hair-clip. When I come out of the room standing barefoot, with my curls already possessing the electrocuted monster look after this long day, a fuzzy-looking Gary is awake and Jeff is talking to him.

"Hey, buddy. I am going to care for you tonight," Jeff says.

Is that a smile on Gary's face? I can't see a thing without my glasses, which are in the car. As I try to squint to see him, the nurse's assistant – the P.C.A. – comes in. All I can tell is he is big. All I want to do is run over and hug Gary. But I'm afraid of tripping and damaging whatever they're trying to hook up. In this get-up with the guys working, I don't think I'd make it to Gary's bed without falling. Instead, I feel my way along the desk to the covers of my make-shift bed and listen to their conversation.

"Hi, I'm Cliff. I'm the P.C.A. I work with Jeff a lot. You're in good hands," he says directly to Gary.

Gary perks up. I hear it in his voice. "You guys going to be here all night?"

I am thrilled to hear his voice. He sounds great. But I don't want to interrupt their conversation.

"Yes, we'll be coming in whenever you need us. If you're in pain, just push the pump," Jeff says. He picks up the white canister with the little red button on top. I think that's what he does, anyway. He pushes it once and I hear a beep. He explains that it beeps when it dispenses the morphine. You can't overdose on the medication because it won't dispense more than a specific amount. He gives it to Gary to push as well. Then he tells Gary to push it six more times. There is no beep. Gary says, "OK, I can't overdo this. I get it."

"We will wake you up every four hours for your vitals. Hope you don't mind," Jeff says.

"Nope, I'm used to it." Gary sounds like an old-timer. He's seems to be acting cool as Jeff seems to check his bandages. They exchange remarks, like how girls like a guy's scars. Gary seems to be enjoying the male bonding. As they talk, I feel the soft pillow on my head and close my eyes because I can't see a thing anyway. The men spend some more time with Gary. I don't remember them leaving.

I feel like I've gotten my own dose of morphine. For the first night in days I sleep soundly. Come morning, though, the residents wake me up with a light show and lack of voice volume control. As they prod Gary's tummy I can tell he is groggy. So am I. I wonder how Gary is doing. There are so many fuzzy figures over him, I figure I'll just wait to ask them. They seem really intense peering over the incision. They mention something about infection and watching for spreading redness. Jeff comes into the room while the residents take Gary's data points. I realize I never heard a machine beep the entire night. That's incredible. I'm sure the night nurses made sure to refill bags before the machine beeped. Jeff is checking the monitors or maybe even checking up on the residents. I'm not sure. Gary goes back to sleep.

"Is he OK?" I ask Jeff.

"Yes. He had a good night. I hope you did too," Jeff says.

"I did. I didn't hear you or the machines once. Thank you."

Jeff sticks around. "The first couple of days post-op, the nurse has fewer patients, so we can focus better," he explains.

I tell him I'm glad. I sit up in my make-shift bed and try to twirl my frizz into a pony tail. "Is Gary still sleeping?"

"Uh huh. He'll sleep most of the day. He won't remember much."

"How is he going to go to the bathroom," I ask. That's been such a big event for him.

"Oh, he has a catheter in him. He won't have to get up." Jeff seems to be checking on the bags. He lets me know his shift is almost over, but he'll be back tonight.

As the day rolls on, I discover the day after surgery is a waiting game. Wait for Gary to wake up. Wait to see if his temperature rises. Wait to see if the incision develops an infection. Wait for the doctor to arrive. It's a test of my patience and I'm not used to so much time. I can't hit a fast-forward button. I appreciate watching Gary rest comfortably. The only place I want to be is by his side. They say he'll be here almost another week and I don't plan to leave. But sitting and waiting is not my strength. I fear that the combination for me of so much alone time, lack of sleep and worry will get me down. I don't want to become depressed, but this sure seems to be the prescription to get me there! I need to stay strong and be ready to question. I've seen how doctors follow protocol, which protects *them*. I need to be Gary's advocate. So, to stay strong I'll look for process improvements in the hospital and start my spa routine. I know that might sound preposterous, but that's where my comfort level is.

This place will make me stronger, just like I told Gary it would.

What You Can Do Now

1. Stock your overnight bag when you head to the hospital.
Be sure to include the basics plus:

    a) Shampoo and conditioner

    b) Slippers and/or socks – there are lots of germs on the floor

    c) Chargers for computers, phones

    d) An outfit you feel professional wearing, for example, business casual. It is a place of business.

    e) Money for the cafeteria

2. Help your loved one feel like they have some control.
Let them make choices. Provide two options. This helps them feel less like a victim of circumstance. If there is really only one choice, like with Gary's surgery delay, make up a second option. If they pick the "pretend" option, have them list the pros and cons of each option. Let them tell you why the real option is better. It may seem like a lot of extra work but the patient will feel some control, leading to a better disposition.

3. Accept the fact that the some of the processes seem redundant.
Yes, the nurses and the residents seem to ask the same questions. Yes, it seems like there is an opportunity for efficiency improvement. But complaining won't get you better care.

4. Help your loved one not feel guilty about needing so much of your attention.
I made recovery time a spa week. I convinced Gary I would finally have lots of extra time and could finally focus on his health and mine.

5. Forget the barking drill-sergeant technique.
I found when I heard myself barking commands I typically didn't get the response I desired. You have to work with what you

have. Use a supportive voice that helps the patient figure out how to help himself. Ask questions to get a sense of their perspective. Sometimes the patient will say, "I don't know." That is the first step for them to come to you for advice. Make suggestions and not orders.

6. Take as much of the doctor's time as you need to gain clarity about the upcoming procedure.

Before you sign the consent form ask for a doctor to review it with you. I was too overwhelmed to do this and didn't really understand the operation. Ask about his record of performance for this type of procedure. Be specific. For example, "In your last 10 operations, what was your complication rate? How many patients needed follow-up surgery within three months?" If you uncover issues or evasiveness, and are not comfortable, find another surgeon. Following the procedure, ask the doctor what he or she actually did. Take notes. Create your own documentation. Include the doctor's summary about how this surgery went compared to other procedures, as well as what the doctor identified as the biggest hurdle and how it was handled. Write down expectations for the recovery process and expected milestones.

* * *

Chapter 8
Spa-Week and Enlightenment

Day One of Spa Week! Gary sleeps and I dash down to the cafeteria, grabbing an oatmeal with caffeine-free tea to go. I consider running up and down the stairs a few times but I really want to give Gary a hug and see how he's feeling and I know the elevator will return me to the room faster. When I open the door to the room, Gary is still asleep. The day nurse turns off a beeping monitor. I walk up to Gary and kiss his forehead. I touch his hand. Nothing stirs him. He looks good though. The nurse reminds me that he'll sleep for most of the next couple of days.

Without losing a beat, the nurse hands me a plastic contraption with a bright blue ball in it. It looks like a toy, with a spout to blow into and gradient like a measuring cup. The nurse explains that in order to avoid pneumonia, Gary must blow into this contraption multiple times a day and try to get the ball to a level 300. It's clear she'd like this to be my job to work with Gary. I guess if the parent is not here then the nurse has to work with the child. But I am glad to be on the team.

Our roles are becoming clearer to me. The hospital staff's job is to get the patient physically better. They've done it over and over and have their system down pat. It is a high volume, transaction-based business model. I enjoy watching people implement consistent processes. This helps reduce error rates and increase thru-put. Every four hours, they measure vitals, food intake and urine outputs, plus gauge the disposition of the patient. Tracking numbers provides indicators for crisis situations. This way, they can see trends, spot concern areas and proactively identify cases needing additional attention. After all, not every case will go smoothly. Just like in corporate America, it's a numbers game. While the data-gathering might make a person feel like a widget, I find the nurses' attention to detail feels like a hug. In my view, the nurses might be chasing the machines, but for the most part they smile as they turn the sound off and sincerely ask how Gary is feeling. That part is not typical in corporate America.

Here's my take on hospital hierarchy: The doctors set the goal, the nurses convey it to me and teach me what to do and then it's in my hands to help my son execute. The implementation process seems to be the same no matter the goal. The goals can range from breathing in a tube to getting the ball to level 300, to walking within 24 hours after surgery, to drinking eight ounces of barium. The nurses seem to appreciate a parent's help. The hospitals don't coach you on how to handle your child, nor should they. The medical staff knows what the widget needs. It is up to the patient to perform or risk the hospital's "Plan B" route. The hospital does have back-up plans if a loved one is unable to motivate the patient to reach expectations. Like, for children who don't drink the barium willingly, the nurses shove an NG tube up the child's nose and into his stomach. You hear kids screaming in this place all day long, which can potentially traumatize the child and the parent. I don't want to know the back-up plan if Gary doesn't blow into this tube.

I pick up the ball contraption and blow into it myself. I hit 300 easily. The nurse comments that it won't be so easy for Gary initially, but he'll get there. I look down at him as I hold the canister and realize I am literally and figuratively holding the ball.

I'm up for another Mother Challenge. While I don't think blowing into this contraption is as disgusting as drinking barium, I'm afraid the challenge might be tougher because Gary might be in too much pain to sit up. His belly seems all cut up. I can't yell at Gary to blow into the darn thing; even when I want something simple done like emptying the dishwasher, yelling doesn't work. It certainly will be a failed tactic to try when he is just waiting for his next morphine hit. But another risk is imminent: pneumonia.

Gary starts to stir from his long sleep. His eyes flutter open and his first action is to hit the morphine pump. The machine beeps and he blinks up at me. The sun shines on his face. He wipes his eyes, almost annoyed by the light intrusion. I stand blocking the sunbeam, but keep the blinds open. The daylight is the best clock around and we need some semblance of time. I kiss his forehead.

As Gary lies here hooked up to the machines, I am terrified things might get worse. Pneumonia? My gut reaction is to tell him to breathe into the machine, right now. He's been post-op 14 hours already and has not breathed once into this contraption. He is finally awake and I am so excited to see him. I don't want him to know I am nervous about complications. Yet, I know we should get started. But I try to hold myself back. After all, he just woke up.

I take a deep breath. The calmer I am, the better. "Good to see you, honey! The doctor said you did great! Nice sleep. How are you feeling?" It all comes out like I am Speedy Gonzalez. He smiles at me and whispers, "Mom, do me a favor and don't ask that question. You know the answer." It's not said snotty, but realistically.

A stupid question, I know. But I don't know what I'm supposed to say. I just want him better. Just two weeks ago, like other moms, I was asking my son about the PSATs and school stuff. I was trying to balance a job and schlepping the kids around. Now, I'm on pneumonia prevention and afraid to tell Gary that this could get worse. After all, he just woke up, seven inches of intestines have been removed plus his appendix and some other body parts I've never heard of. But, my challenge is to get him breathing up to 300. Tomorrow they want him walking around the floor. For me, this is harder than hitting goals in corporate America. But I have to try.

"Gary, the nurse mentioned when you were sleeping that you'll need to blow into this pump to help your lungs. She wants you to hit the 300 mark."

"Huh?" Gary groans.

He's tired and not focused. He falls right back to sleep. He's not going to blow into it now. I'll let him rest and we'll try again later. I take out my laptop to write some more about our experience. The trip to the E.R. seems centuries ago even though it's been less than a week. Eventually, I notice Gary stirring again. I look at my watch and three hours have passed. Gary's not taken a single breath in the pump and it's almost lunch time. The word pneumonia echoes as a refrain in my head. The nurse mentioned on her last vitals check that Gary's temperature was slightly elevated. My nerves are raw.

Gary stirs and hits the morphine pump before he looks up at me. I get up from the couch and walk over to him. I kiss his forehead and this time I do not ask how he is feeling.

"Good to see you," I say.

"Yeah," he says.

"How about I make a log for you so you can show the doctor how you are succeeding with the pump? Dr. Carroll said he will stop by today." I hold up the contraption.

"Huh?" Gary looks at it quizzically.

"How about I leave the pump on the table by your bed? You'll just need to blow into it and record the result. Then you can show it to Dr. Carroll," I say.

"OK" tumbles out. I know he'll try to impress the doctor, not me.

I move the pump to the bed and write on a piece of paper:

Time	Height of Balls

I hold back from saying, "Want to make the first recording?" I want to say it so bad.

I continue instead with, "Dr. Carroll mentioned trying every hour. I'm not sure when he's coming today. It's almost noon. He could be here soon." OK, am I so much of a manipulating mother? What am I supposed to do? He has to blow in this thing!

Gary takes his hand and touches the button to raise the head portion of his bed. He winces a little as the bed rises.

"Mom, move the table closer, please."

I follow his directions. He picks up the pump and tries to blow hard. It looks like it takes all his strength. The ball slowly starts to rise but it does not go very far. Gary takes another breath and tries again. He seems spent.

"Mom, I got a 150. I'll get it higher next time. Let me write it down."

My smile feels as if it travels from inside my heart onto my face. Gary looks at me but says nothing. He writes down the time and score on the paper. I know he'll start to track this himself now. I decide to let this victory sink in and not mention tomorrow's challenge – walking. Instead I ask Gary if he'd mind if I grab some lunch to go in the cafeteria.

"Nope," he says.

"You want to watch some TV," I ask.

"Nope. Just go, Mom. I'll be OK," he says and he seems to nod off.

I feel a little light-hearted for the first time in days. My Gary's drive is still there. I stroll to the elevator. A dad walks toward his child's room. Feeling more confident and grateful that Gary will be getting better, I try to spread some of my positive energy. I say hello to the dad. Just like the uncle of boy with the brain injury, I ask, "How is your child doing?"

"Well, she has Crohn's disease and it's her 15th surgery. *She's 19.*"

I feel like someone has hit me in the head with a two-by-four! The dad continues so fast toward his child's room he clearly does not want to talk. I don't know what to do. I want to learn more. I want to say I'm sorry. Will this be our life? I thought the surgery corrected the disease? I don't know other parents of Crohn's kids and I want to seem supportive. I've discovered my inner strength is my key coping mechanism, so I figure maybe it can help him too. As he races toward his daughter's room, I blurt out, "I pray for you to have the strength to help your daughter."

With those words he stops dead in his tracks. He turns around. He looks directly at me. He takes a couple of steps towards me. Maybe he wants to chat after all or maybe he wants to slug me. He says, "I am already strong. This is hell." Then he turns around and races off.

I feel like a total fool. Who am I to think it's my place to help someone try to feel better? I wish I'd kept my mouth shut. The elevator doors close on my foolishness. Fifteen surgeries? I can't believe Gary could be back here again. I don't even want to think about it. I walk listlessly to the cafeteria, my head down as I select the lettuce for my salad. A perky woman in her 40's with blondish hair is also grabbing a salad. She has a bottle of water on her tray and no dessert. Maybe she is on the spa diet too. With my foot-in-mouth disease, I stare at the salad dressing instead of talking to her.

She asks me, "How long have you been in the hospital?"

I look up. She is smiling. I must look dejected. "About a week. My son had surgery on Tuesday." Since she started the conversation, I figure it's safe to ask, "How about you?" In the outside world, I am used to the typical exchange of "How are you?" Here, I guess the key question to ask is, "How long?"

"My son had emergency surgery on Monday," she says. "He has Crohn's disease."

"Was it by Dr. Carroll?" I inquire.

"Yes. How'd you know?"

"Well, my son's surgery was postponed because of an emergency case," I say. "I guessed. Your son? How is he doing?"

"OK. We're waiting for him to pass gas and have a bowel movement before he's released," she says. Parents of kids with G.I. issues, including myself, tend to be comfortable discussing shit with strangers.

"Me too!" I exclaim like a child. Her easy smile makes me think she can help me understand more about the disease. "Do you have a moment to eat lunch here?"

"Sure," she says walking to get some utensils.

I choose a table against a back wall, where it's quiet and I sit down and wait. I look around and realize there seems to be a pecking order in the cafeteria. It's sort of like the pink and orange flamingos I've seen in the San Diego Zoo. While the flamingos are all in the same exhibit, they stand on opposite sides of the watering hole based on their color. Here, the "white coats" seem to be the dividing line in the cafeteria, with the doctors on one side and the residents on the other. The patients' families are scattered in between. I wave to my new acquaintance so she can easily find me behind the white coats and I realize the cliché really is true: Birds of a feather flock together. I have a battery of questions for her, like when was her son diagnosed, what medications is he on, is he behind in school, how much pain does he have, but before I get to bombard her she blurts out, "This is real hard on my other son. My husband and I keep rotating being here. Our younger one misses family time."

"I have two sons, too!" I'm overly enthusiastic, as if I am trying to maximize commonality so we can become fast friends.

She continues, "My other son is autistic. He needs routine and this is really hard for him. My husband is too tired to have the patience he needs." She nibbles her salad.

She has one with Crohn's, which triggers crippling stomach pains in between diarrhea runs, and the other child is autistic; I bet she needs this lunch-time chat more than I do. I hold back on my questions and she continues, "We both work and my husband feels guilty if he doesn't get to the hospital but he needs to pick up Sean, my other son. I just want to take Andy home tomorrow. I hope he poops today."

"Me too," I say, meaning both of our sons.

I really want to ask her about Crohn's. She really needs to talk about autism. I try very hard to be a good listener. She says how Sean tends to be in his own world a lot. He gets overly excited and has trouble focusing in school. It sounds like he has a pretty intense challenge. I nod as if I am listening but I really want to talk about Crohn's. As she talks, she doesn't appear sorry for herself. She doesn't question why her family has both kids with tough medical issues, not aloud, anyway. She seems to accept her plight as a mother and just wants to help her kids get the best care possible. I'm fascinated, because, deep down I'm still hoping Gary can keep up with the other kids at school.

Before Gary got sick, I remember lunches with other moms during which we'd discuss high school course selection so we could help our kids be on the right track for a good college. I remember at one lunch a mom with a child a few years ahead of Gary was disappointed because her child was getting a "C" in an Advanced Placement course. She spent the whole lunch consumed with finding out if I knew a tutor, evaluating if this would ruin his future college choices, and then complained about how she thought the child was lazy. The mom seemed really disappointed in her child, as if his performance were a reflection of her.

School performance seems to be the last thing on my new friend's mind. The more she talks the more I can see she just loves her kids for who they are. I feel more comfortable with her than some of my previous lunch buddies in town.

"Do you have a moment to stop up and meet my son Andy?" she says.

"Sure," I say, hoping that he and Gary will get better, become friends, and reach their dreams. Gary seems to find a lot of support from his friends from the Crohn's camp he went to last summer. I bet this child would fit in with that crew. They have the same feathers, after all.

As we go up in the elevator, I tell her my name and she shakes my hand. Her name is Cathy. I motion to turn right so I can walk by Gary's room first just to see how he is doing. I've been gone longer than I expected. I peek in and he is asleep. Cathy says Andy's room is a few doors down. I wonder how she is coping with two children with chronic health issues and appears not to be a basket case. She waves to the nurse on the floor and smiles easily at other parents in the hall.

We pass a room with a pretty teenage girl with long straight brown hair who is reading a book in bed. She is not hooked up to any monitors and looks physically healthy to me. There is a person sitting outside her door, just staring all day and night. I suspect she is on suicide watch. I've still not seen the girl's parents.

When we pass the room, Cathy says you never really know what's happening inside people's homes. She says something about even if you think you have it bad, someone has it worse. We continue walking toward Andy's room.

Andy's room looks just like Gary's – same bed, TV and desk – predictable, just like hotel rooms. Andy is lying in bed hooked up to monitors similar to Gary's. But his head and arms are jerking from side to side. He looks like the paraplegic that goes to Gary's school. Sometimes when I am waiting on the school pick-up line, I see the boy being raised in his wheelchair on a platform onto a special school bus. I always try not to stare. It takes three adults to transfer him at the end of the day. I look directly at Andy and try to conceal my shock. I walk right up to the side of his bed, like nothing is wrong.

"Hi, I'm Randi. My son had the same surgery as you," I say.

He cannot talk, apparently, but he smiles at me. I can see it in between head wobbles. He hears me!

Cathy whispers to me that he understands what is said to him.

He just can't talk. He can make loud sounds if he needs attention. She then tells Andy that we will be outside in the hall. She smiles at him and him back to her. I take a "moment memory" snapshot. In the past, I would have thought this was awful and a totally depressing situation, but I see that new color I'd never noticed before I came to this children's hospital. It fills the entire space and it makes me feel alive.

In the hall, Cathy tells me Andy has cerebral palsy. She seems grateful that I treated him just like another kid. She tells me that since he can't talk, she has no idea what he has been feeling with this disease. Maybe she can talk to Gary and he can help her.

She asks me, "Do you think Gary can visit him?"

"Like a play-date? Why not? He's not walking yet but he will be soon. I'm sure he'll want to stop by," I say.

I sense she wants me to know more about her story. I failed with that father an hour and a half ago but I seem to have passed this test with Cathy. She leans up against the wall and continues, "Andy was supposed to be born at this hospital but there were complications during my labor. I was too trusting and naïve to question the doctors. Besides, I was in labor. I remember this young doctor on staff that night and I guess he did not know what to do." She pauses. "I should have insisted right away on a more experienced doctor. They ended up Medevacking me to Boston Children's for the birth, but in the meantime Andy lost too much oxygen. He would have been a healthy child," she says. My heart breaks for this woman.

"My husband doesn't like this place. When Andy needed emergency surgery on Monday, we had no choice but to bring him here. Now, I just want Andy to poop so we can all go home."

Oh my friggin' goodness, this poor family. This time, I know saying "I am praying for you to have the strength to cope" is a mistake. "I'm sorry you've had to go through this," I say. I take her hand and hold it. She doesn't pull away. Maybe I am learning what to say after all.

She says, "Can I meet your son?"

"Sure, he just had surgery yesterday, though. He's been sleeping a lot."

Cathy tells Andy she'll be back real soon and we head off to visit Gary. I see a nurse in our room taking vitals. On the paper Gary has made another recording. Gary's bed is raised. He is sitting up. I am so excited to see him. He smiles when I enter the room but before I can say anything the nurse announces how he is doing great. I beam. He beams. Before lunch I was feeling sorry for myself. Now I'm feeling sorry for Cathy. Cathy introduces herself to Gary and says her son had similar surgery.

Gary tells her, "It's only been a day but I feel so much better already. I bet your son does too."

"I hope so. Will you visit us?"

"Sure. I plan on starting to try to walk tomorrow. I bet after a few tries I can make it to his room," Gary says.

"Well, if Andy doesn't poop tonight we will still be here. I'll stop by tomorrow to see how you are doing," Cathy says.

"Great," Gary says as Cathy leaves the room. I decide not to tell him, yet, about her son. I'm still shocked. Gary points to the record of his breathing tube. The latest recording says 200.

I look at Gary and I think about Cathy's son. I feel weak-kneed. I'm not used to such large doses of perspective. I start to cry, not a little. Suddenly, I can't catch my breath. I don't know how her son blew into the contraption. How do they do it? I've never met anyone like her or maybe I've never taken the time to really find out about anyone like her. Gary is staring at me crying. He lets me have my moment. He probably thinks I am all *faklempt* about him blowing into the tube.

In corporate America, I spent an inordinate amount of time on "busy work." How many midnight e-mails did I write? I even felt sort of proud; my manager could see the time I was working. Image was a key part of success. Luckily, I am not there now, because I'd have to put my best face forward and hide my true reality. I remember when my dad was in the hospital and I was sending e-mails sitting next to his hospital bed. On maternity leave, I even negotiated a contract while breast-feeding Matt. If I couldn't keep up, I would be labeled a performance problem and the piranhas would eat me alive. I knew so many people who got laid off, but never really grasped what might have been happening in their personal lives.

With that daily grind so far away, I feel I can see more clearly now. Something about the hospital makes life so real, so clear about what is important. It's not about Gary's A's in biology, or getting into the best college or increasing my sales volume. That's the busy work. Those things are designed to increase earning power. But I can't purchase a truly beautiful life, though maybe I could buy the image of one. A wonderful life, for me, I realize, is built on turning the moments I get into great memories for me and my loved ones.

I take a deep breath, pull myself together, walk right up to him and kiss Gary on the forehead. Gary picks up the contraption and takes another breath into the tube. I don't know how far the ball goes, but it's one small breath for him and a great life insight for me.

Dr. Carroll comes into the room. I grab another tissue and try to discretely wipe my face. I bet my mascara has run down my cheek. At least my hair is not frizzed out. If it were, I'd look like the maid from The Rocky Horror Picture show. Dr. Carroll goes over to Gary, who is sitting up and seems happy to see the doctor. Gary points at his sheet with his scores.

"Wow, you've been busy. Good. How are you feeling?" the doctor asks.

Gary says, "I have no pain when I am peeing." I guess that's an answerable question for the doctor, but not a mom! Then Gary says, "How *am* I peeing, anyway?"

"You have a catheter inserted in your penis. It will be there a few days," Dr. Carroll says.

"Oh, I didn't want that," Gary says. "But you know what? It

doesn't hurt to pee. It's great. Thank you."

"Can I take a look at your belly?" the doctor asks, and Gary says sure.

Gary lies flat on the bed and Dr. Carroll lifts Gary's hospital gown and inspects the incision. I peek at it as well. It's about the same length and place as my Caesarean scar. With a bathing suit, no one will ever know it's there. There are three other little bandages, but Dr. Carroll seems to be focusing on the main one.

"You see that little redness?" he says to me. I nod my head and he continues, "We have to make sure it doesn't spread." Dr. Carroll takes out a ball point pen and draws a circle around the redness. The black ink mark seems so elementary to me after such a complicated surgery. I always tell my kids not to write on themselves, but clearly it's not really a big deal. What *would* be is an infection. And pneumonia. And I'm still wondering if they're going to put him on some toxic medicine for maintenance or if he can go back to nutritional therapy.

I say to the doctor, "You mentioned last night you took out the diseased intestines. Will Gary be able to continue nutritional therapy?" This is my main concern. I really want to help Gary avoid some of the medicines because I know some of them may cause lymphoma in later years.

"That is a question for your G.I. Has he been here yet?"

"Not yet."

"Oh, he'll be here. I was able to do this laparoscopically," Dr. Carroll says, admiring his work.

I guess it's not his job to figure out how Gary will keep his pipes working. The surgeon proceeds to tell Gary about the operation. I take out the crumpled paper diagram and give it to him. The doctor goes through the same speech I already heard. I am just staring at Gary. He seems like his old self, interested, engaged and wanting to learn. Dr. Carroll mentions that he'll be back again tomorrow and to just keep blowing into the tube and maybe even to try to sit on the side of the bed today.

After Dr. Carroll leaves, I walk over to Gary. I want to see the pen mark. It's pretty red inside the border, like someone colored it. I just hope the color stays in the lines. A rapid knock on the door startles me. Could it be Dr. Stark again? Ah, no, it's Dr. Simmon, Gary's G.I. Thank goodness – the plumber who cares for the pipes! I haven't really talked to him since our airplane chat. He'll be Gary's doctor through college and I want to make sure he knows I am not mad at him (just at Dr. Stark, the one who put Gary on the steroids). Instead of rehashing the whole thing, I take another tack.

"Dr. Simmon, it's so good to see you." I smile broadly. "Dr. Carroll said Gary did great!"

"I know. It looks like they got out all of the Crohn's disease," he says, professionally.

"I know, they took out a lot of stuff," I say as I pick up the crumpled piece of paper. "Let me tell you about it. Let me know if I understood the operation."

He nods his head and pulls up a chair.

"I don't remember the name of the operation. It's real long. But, I can tell you on the diagram what Dr. Carroll did."

Dr. Simmon says, "Gary developed a fistula, a typical complication of Crohn's. His appendix attached to his bladder causing a hole that filled with fluid. They did an ileocecectomy."

"Oh yeah, that is it. When the doctor described it earlier he said he'd cut out two inches of small intestine and five inches of large intestine..." I point to the diagram. "Then he removed the appendix that was on Gary's bladder causing a hole. He sewed up the bladder and removed the ileum and scrotum." I say it practically in one breath and Dr. Simmon giggles.

"It's amazing how much you got. But Gary's scrotum? Are you sure?" Dr. Simmon says.

"Oh, yes, the scrotum *and* the ileum they are gone plus even the appendix. Dr. Carroll took them out." I say it with confidence.

Dr. Simmon laughs louder. "I hope he didn't do that." He looks at me.

I think about what he's saying. Suddenly I'm horrified! I hope Gary still has his scrotum! I stumble around my embarrassment and Dr. Simmon is gentleman enough not to humiliate me. I say, "So, what did he take out?"

"The cecum." He looks at Gary. "You'll be able to have children. Don't worry."

Gary lifts the blanket and examines what's underneath. "Mom, I'm all there." He breaks out in a wide grin and rolls his eyes. We all erupt in full belly laughter.

I pause for a moment-memory-shot of Gary and Dr. Simmon and me cracking up. Maybe this leg of the trip won't be so bad after all.

What You Can Do Now

---

1. Become a nurse helper.

Learn what the expectations are and help your loved one hit the goals. Find out what needs to occur post-op, like blowing into the ball contraption and how many walks a day the patient should take.

2. Keep a record of a loved one's accomplishments.

If possible let the patient record their progress. Let everyone see how well they are doing.

3. Go to any meetings for family members.

Sometimes the hospital will hold a special breakfast for the loved ones. This is the best opportunity to listen and learn from others.

4. Understand the roles of the surgeon versus your doctor.

Who determines aftercare? Do they agree on the goals of the surgery? Repeat back what you think they did. Let them correct you. Ask for the information in writing.

* * *

Chapter 9
The Other "Guests"

The days after surgery seem to blend into each other. With no clocks on the walls, only the light streaming into Gary's room hints toward the time of day. That, and the residents' rounds before dawn, which become my automatic alarm clock (one that lacks a much-needed snooze button). Except for early morning rounds, nothing appears to have a schedule. Doctors pop in and out randomly, nurses stop by periodically and meals are eaten when the patient is awake. It's a stark contrast to my time in corporate America, when my days were booked to the minute with meetings and travel plans, and I could tell you what I'd be doing next Tuesday at 2:30 p.m. Yet, now I have no memory of what was so critical that I used to take a daily Tums to calm my stomach. Whatever goals I did achieve do not seem as significant as my days here. Each day I help Gary grow stronger. I've taken moment-memory shots here in the hospital of the first time he sat up in bed, the first time he stood on the floor and the first time the blue ball hit 300. Each time we high-fived each other. My new perspective is a prescription for calming my nerves.

Some moment memories aren't so great though. With the door to the room open, I keep seeing a boy, 9-ish, with a big round head, tugging a nurse's hand and stalking the halls. He's screaming, "Where's Mommy?" The boy's head is immense, maybe big as a basketball. It looks like it's filled with fluid, taut like a water balloon. Gary's been here over a week, and in this time we've never seen the mom. But I hear these relentless yells at least three times a day. Even I feel like yelling, "Get here already!" The poor boy becomes so belligerent; the poor nurse can't seem to settle him down. I feel bad for the nurse and the boy.

The teenage girl is still here, too. She sits in her bed, with the door wide open as the "sitter," a hospital worker, stares at her every move. The patient has no privacy; this way she can't hurt herself. From what I can tell, her parents have not been back since the day she checked in. These kids' moment memories are my constant reminders to make sure my son's memories of this place are not horror pictures.

Cathy and I visit each other every day as our children wait for the big poop. Today, Gary plans on meeting Cathy's son since Gary can now walk to the other side of the floor. Before we venture out, I tell Gary about Andy's cerebral palsy. I explain that Andy understands what is being said to him. Gary mentions that he's seen kids in school like this. He tells me it's not a big deal. It's said without the eye roll. I don't tell him that Cathy says it's the hospital's fault, due to the circumstances during her labor.

"I want to meet him, Mom. I can tell Cathy what he's going through with the surgery. Let's go now," he says, sounding like a man.

Gary asks me to unplug his monitors. (They have battery backup.) I drape the power cord over the silver pole holding the beeping machines. Since they took out the catheter the other day, it's become my job to squeeze behind the bed and unplug the equipment to give Gary the freedom to walk. The first time I unplugged him, he chose to walk into the bathroom. Not a far trek, but a key one. It had been days since he used a bathroom. He closed the door. I listened for the screams and I heard nothing. I even walked up to the door to check if I could hear anything. It sounded like Niagara Falls in there but with no cursing. I couldn't believe it. Then I heard a huge "WOW" louder than any previous curse. The door knob turned and I scurried to the sink and acted nonchalant as Gary exited.

"Mom, it doesn't hurt to pee. It's amazing."

After a couple of days, Gary mastered walking the whole floor without stopping. Now the small trek a couple of doors down is easy.

"I can practically sprint this," he says as he rolls the monitor to his right.

I realize this is the first time Gary seems able to walk and focus beyond himself. In the past he'd stare at the floor and take small steps. Now he's taking in the scenery. Gary sees the sitter outside the teenage girl's room with the door open. As usual, the sitter doesn't even read a book. She just stares at the teenage girl in the room.

"What's up with that?" Gary asks me, as if he's hanging out with a friend and seeing something weird.

"I think she tried to kill herself. Now she is not left alone," I say.

"Really?" He says it like he is truly stumped.

"Sometimes emotional pain is just as tough as physical," I say, repeating Cathy's comments about the girl.

Gary pauses outside her room and glances inside. The sitter does not turn around to see him. She doesn't take her eye off the girl who is in the same position as I always see her, sitting on her bed reading a book. The girl doesn't look up either. The room seems stark.

"There are no cards in there," Gary whispers to me.

I just nod and start us walking again.

"I love the cards from the kids back home hanging up in my room. They make me feel special. I think I'll always send a card now when someone is in the hospital," Gary says.

I just nod but inside I am *kvelling*. This Yiddish word means feeling so proud from the inside out. Somehow this place is teaching us so much.

We arrive at Andy's room. It's a similar set-up to Gary's. Andy's has a few cards and no flowers or stuffed animals. There's just Cathy, his vibrant mom, who beams as she opens the door. It's a real play-date for the boys.

"Welcome! We're so glad you're here," she says.

"Me too!" I say. I flash back to when Gary was three. I loved play-dates because I got time to be with another mom. I'd just hope the kids played quietly so we could share a pot of tea and a few minutes of peace and gossip. A week ago, I was afraid that Gary wouldn't be able to relate to kids his own age. His experiences were so different and I resented it. I can't imagine what I would have thought then about his "play-date" with a paraplegic. Gary pulls along his pole and walks over to Andy's monitors. Andy looks up at Gary. His head bobs back and forth but I can tell he is really trying to look at him.

"Hi. My name is Gary. We had the same surgery. Man, I know you were hurting." He smiles so warmly as he says it.

Andy smiles back. They have something in common and instead of me wanting them to play by themselves so we can have a break, I just want to watch them interact. I look at Cathy, whose eyes are tearing up. I put my arm around her and squeeze.

Gary says, "I don't see the catheter bag by your bed. I bet you love that." Andy flails but it looks like a happy flailing. "You see this monitor? It is checking your oxygen level. It says 97 – great," Gary says, looking directly at Andy.

Gary continues, "This one is for giving you the medication. Guess what? It's perfect." He says it with such authority that I well up just like Cathy. Cathy squeezes my hand. Gary looks over the rest of the monitors and says, "I bet you are gonna go home soon. Your mom said you are like me – just waiting for the poop."

Andy's hand seems to fly up, conveying, "Yeah man."

Gary smiles at him and says, "Want to race?"

Andy keeps his gaze on Gary.

"OK, let's see who poops first and gets out of this joint," Gary challenges. Maybe all boys like a little competition because Andy's face turns red. He looks like he is trying to push out a poop that instant to win.

"Hey, it has to come naturally. Don't force it," Gary says.

A nurse drops in the room to check some of Andy's bags hanging on the machine. She makes it before it starts to beep. She wins the round. As the nurse starts checking the fluid levels, the three of us go out to the hall. Once Cathy is away from the door so Andy can't hear, Cathy seems thrilled to finally find a translator.

She says to Gary, "I could tell he was in pain. What was it like?"

"Know what? I bet he feels so much better now. The surgery is a miracle. I'm starting to forget the pain. The most important thing is you're here." His voice sounds deep, like a man's. But Gary's simplicity puts a huge smile on Cathy's face. To think at 15 he already knows what to say to parents and I, at 47, am still learning.

The nurse comes out of the room and tells us Andy pooped.

Gary runs in the room. "You won, man!"

Jubilation erupts. Without losing a beat, Cathy picks up Andy's already packed bag and looks for a discharge nurse.

We don't exchange e-mail addresses. We both know our lives are hectic enough without saying platitudes that will never come to fruition, like "Let's do lunch." Cathy wishes Gary and me the best as she readies the wheelchair. Gary high-fives Andy, who looks like he won the biggest game of his life.

I stroll back to the room, watching Gary walk in his hospital gown and rubber-bottomed socks, pushing the silver pole holding the machines. I feel so happy for Cathy and Andy. Pooping means his system is working. We pass the boy with the big head and I wave hello to him. He stops screaming and waves back. I see the Indian mom wheeling her son in the hall and I wave to them as well. The boy smiles at us and the mom waves. His head does not tilt as much; he is getting stronger. It's so strange. Just last week, I was feeling sorry for myself because my child was in pain and exposed to such sorry situations. Yet, as my new neighbors respond to me, I feel a sense of joy that I rarely felt in my past harried days racing between conference rooms and endless meetings.

Now, I have all day to chat. It's a new me. In my corporate past when I was scheduled to the minute, I could barely breathe. Days flew by. Here there are no formal times for appointments. I wave to people in the halls. We wait for the doctors to fit us in their schedule and show up. Back in my corporate days, I mostly thought about what I had to do next and how to avoid the next layoff. To me, that was like a life or death situation. Here, I haven't needed to take a single Tums.

Back in the room, Gary takes a nap and I think about how to keep him out of here forever. I spy Dr. Stark heading down the hall. It has been a couple of days since she stared me down in the cafeteria. I recoil, like a mouse peeking out of the hole and sensing danger. A couple of minutes later, I hear her rapid knocks as she bursts into Gary's room. In the same time it takes for the door to open, her face transforms from serious to happy-go-lucky. She has double-gulped the saccharine-infused coffee to sweeten her demeanor from the wolf to a kerchief-wearing sweet grandma, even though she's not that old. The commotion stirs Gary awake. Dr. Stark strides over to Gary's bedside without saying hello to me. "You look great. How are you feeling? Can I touch your belly?" Dr. Stark shoots out the statements in rapid precision.

Gary must be tired by now of each doctor pressing on his stomach. Why do they each take a turn? Shouldn't the doctors just talk to each other? Certainly, the residents this morning noticed he was improving. They all poked his stomach until he was fully awake. Even I can see the redness is not spreading outside the line. I doubt poking it over and over again helps. But what do I know?

I sense there is another reason for her visit. Once she lowers Gary's gown on his belly, she looks up at me sitting on the chair and walks over. The closer she comes toward me, the more I feel that the grandma's kerchief is slipping, revealing her real character. Cornered in my chair, I wait.

She holds up the book I gave her before Gary's surgery, "Breaking the Vicious Cycle" by Elaine Gottschall. I've been told it is the bible for Israelis with Crohn's disease. It gives reasons and recipes for eating certain foods. My friend whose husband is from Israel says many people swear by it even though it's a pretty strict diet, heavy on vegetables, fruits and protein with limited processed foods and sugar. It has to do with limiting foods that bad bacteria like to ingest in the intestine. The medical consensus is that what causes Crohn's disease is unknown, but researchers believe it is the result of an abnormal reaction by the body's immune system. Normally, the immune system protects people from infection by identifying and destroying bad bacteria, viruses, or other potentially harmful foreign substances. Researchers believe that in Crohn's disease the immune system attacks even the bacteria that are harmless or even useful.

I've read that bad bacteria thrive on sugar and complex carbohydrates, like spaghetti and bread. At the same time, there are foods that the bad bacteria don't like, like cayenne pepper, which Gary loves in his chili as a seasoning. A lot has been printed about eating blueberries for antioxidants. I hope that feeding him good foods might help Gary keep his intestines inflammation-free. In the past, when doctors said Gary could eat anything and I wanted him to gain weight, I'd take him to Dunkin' Donuts for hot chocolate and glazed doughnuts. I'd never heard about "bad bacteria." Now I know that doughnuts are a feast for them. Even with his taking 12 Pentasa pills every day, Gary got worse. Maybe the food had an impact. Maybe if I'd kept him off refined sugar, the Pentasa would have worked longer. It got so bad we ended up here. Gottschall's book seems to make sense to me, now.

"I'm familiar with nutritional therapy," Dr. Stark says, as she throws the book on the desk. "I do not support it because there isn't any statistical evidence that it works. Our medicines are tested and the side effects are monitored. There are exhaustive studies on these medicines and I can advise you on their results, but I can't tell you the outcomes of eating anything in particular," she says.

Dr. Stark seems to be aligned with the majority of doctors in the United States who shy away from a dietary approach for Inflammatory Bowel Disease. I just stare at her. This seems bizarre. She is basically saying she will recommend Remicade over nutritional therapy because she knows the chance of getting a lymphoma is small. I've checked out the FDA's website. It says,

"The FDA has completed its analysis of tumor necrosis factor (TNF) blockers and has concluded that there is an increased risk of lymphoma and other cancers associated with the use of these drugs in children and adolescents."[7]

Cancer is a big problem, no matter how small the chance. Dr. Stark seems to feel that patients should eat anything if it agrees with them. The medical journals apparently do not have statistical evidence of food intake and inflammation levels. Unlike pharmaceutical companies, farmers don't tend to spend money studying the medicinal effects of their product.

I'm an engineer, not a nutritionist, but it seems to me that if you have a digestive disorder, food might be an irritant causing inflammation. Instead of debating Dr. Stark and getting bombarded with medical statistics about medicines and figures and terminology that will smother me until I feel overwhelmed, I thank her for returning the book. I think she thinks I'm sincere, like I finally boarded her train. As she walks toward the door, she smiles and I reflect the same smile she gives me. I wonder if it looks as forced as it feels.

Gary asks for his lunch. It's a heap of pasta covered with marinara sauce. Pasta. Something the book says to avoid because it is a complex carbohydrate creating a feast for the bad bacteria. But it's protocol to serve pasta in the hospital as long as the patient hasn't tested positive for gluten sensitivity. They don't follow the book, because it's not scientifically tested and only has testimonials from patients. I watch Gary gorge himself. Marinara sauce drips down from a piece of Gary's spaghetti onto his hospital gown. I say nothing. But I wonder. Gary finishes the meal with a chocolate-frosted fudge brownie for dessert. I'm thrilled he's eating. Gary licks the last of the frosting off of his fingers. I may have lost this battle against flour and sugar but I am not giving up. Eating like everybody else lets Gary feel normal. I am not sure how to change this food path. I'd like to implement a nutritional-based solution rather than fill Gary with toxic drugs. But it is the doctors who have to approve it and Gary who has to live it.

This will be an uphill battle and I'll need allies. The medical community is armed with facts, titles and lots of experience, which is great. I have nothing. I just have a gut instinct and a determination to help my son thrive as naturally as possible despite this disease. Who can help me? I look around the room at all the cards hanging on the walls. It's a glimpse of the people who care about us in our lives. I pick up each card and I visualize the person who sent the card and reread it. For a second, holding their card, I feel like they are giving me a hug. After several cards, I think of some old friends I've supported in the past who might be good on my team, and look to see if they sent a card. There's nothing like being in the hospital to give you time to reflect and assess life. My best recruits are probably on the wall. I have to find people who know the right things to say to support me in helping Gary find a plan when he gets out of here. To develop the core support team, I'll need to make some cuts. I take cards off the wall, eliminating anyone who said, "At least it's not diabetes," or "he's young," or "God only gives you what you can handle." I know they mean well but their justifications only seem unfair. I place these cards on my left side.

Gary isn't paying any attention to me. He falls back to sleep. Cards are strewn all over the desk. I hold up a card and think about the person. Giving true support to a person with a health obstacle is typically above and beyond what most people have experience with, including, fortunately, my friends. I am not surprised not one card has made it to the right-hand pile yet.

As I sort through the cards, I realize I've used hospitalizations before as a barometer for measuring "friendship value." I think this can be a mistake. When I was 29, I was hit by a drunk driver, almost killed, and lay in the hospital with a collapsed lung, three broken ribs and internal bleeding so severe the doctors weren't sure if I'd ever have kids. After a few days in the hospital, when I started to feel a little physically stronger and needed emotional support, I called my friends.

My first call was to Becky, an old friend, someone I'd known since kindergarten. She still looked like she did in her kindergarten class photo, with her big blue eyes and wavy brown hair. Over the years, I listened to her school problems, bullying problems and, when she was in her 20's, the financial woes of her dad. When I called her for support from my hospital bed, the conversation quickly turned to her tale of woe about her father not having a pension and how lucky I was to work for GE and get a pension. I realized I'd spent my time always listening to her, but I never realized that she was incapable of listening to me. That was our last conversation.

I'm not a whiner and never have been. I was in pain and hooked up to a machine blowing air into my lung. But my voice still sounded strong. I called Jake, a college friend. I told him what was going on and when he figured I was done with the update, he told me his sister was getting married and that she'd just bought a four-bedroom house with two-and-a-half bathrooms. He emphasized the half like it was beyond spectacular. I couldn't breathe on my own without the noisy machine and he was just chatting with me like nothing was wrong. That was our last conversation.

I couldn't believe these two. I tried one more. I called Julie, a college friend, with wavy brown hair, big eyes and a vivacious personality. She was someone I'd listened to since freshman year. In the last decade, I knew every professional problem, every boyfriend problem and even her financial troubles as she worked in Manhattan with a foreign language degree. I was touched as she listened to my story for about 10 minutes. Then I spent 40 minutes hearing about her decision to break up with her boyfriend. She never mentioned the loud machine in the background pumping air into my lung, keeping me alive. I didn't dump her, though. Like the others, I realized she didn't know what to say. Maybe I was expecting more than they were capable of giving.

I can't get mad at everyone who doesn't know what to say. It's not their fault; they haven't been touched with a similar experience. I've learned I have to be careful. It had been almost 20 years since my car accident. Since then I've had plenty of time to make new friends. I've focused on adding people into my life who enhance me and support me, not solely drain me. Helping others made me feel good about myself. It still does. But now I look for people who, when in spite of their problems, want to learn new skills to overcome them, not fixate on their past or keep score with stuff.

The next card I pick up is Reena's. She is the one who gave me the book. She also has been organizing dinners for when we return. She said she has enough people wanting to bring over meals that we can go a month without cooking. I place her card on the right side.

I hear a light knock on the door. I put down the next card without looking at the name and I see Beverly. I can't believe she's here. I love Beverly. She's a person I consider my twin from Fairfield. I met her when our kids were in middle school. Besides us both being only children, being married for 21 years, and each having two boys the same ages, we both have technical degrees and are accustomed to working predominantly with men. We think alike. However, if anyone met us, they'd never guess how similar we are. She is from Latin America, has flowing long straight brown hair and speaks with a Spanish accent. But our core values are the same. She even eats healthfully. She taught me to make a Uruguayan green apple and celery salad that Gary loves. As I get up to say hello, I see it's her card next in the pile! I race to the door to give her a big hug.

Standing next to her in the hall is her son, Gill. After middle school our boys found different interests. Gary's veered toward tennis and Gill's toward skateboarding. Despite our kids' preference to hang with different crowds, Beverly and I remain very close. Beverly glances in the door. Gary is asleep. Beverly nods "no." She doesn't want to disturb him. I tell her it's OK, we can sit in the room and we'll see if he wakes up. I'm thinking he'll be as excited as I am to have a visitor. Gill sits on the chair by the desk and seems to stare at Gary sleeping. He fumbles for his cellphone. Beverly and I squeeze next to each other on the couch. She hands me a big bag with tissue paper and ribbons. Excitedly, I pull apart the present to reveal a basket of body and facial lotions. Beverly says it's to enhance my "spa experience" in the hospital. As I unravel the soft pastel shades of tissue paper, I uncover scented bath salts for calming the nerves. There is a lavender moisturizer that the packaging says should bring a sense of peace. It's the perfect gift.

I'm thrilled she brought Gill here to see Gary. But as Gary sleeps through the visit, I realize the truth: I need the visit. I keep making a thousand excuses for my friends not to visit: Gary is resting, they are too busy. I don't think I tell anyone to come. But Beverly knew something I didn't realize, that one real hug, one friendly face would lift my spirits. I parade her and Gill around the floor to introduce them to the nurses. It is like saying, "See, I really have a life. We really are loved." Right before Beverly and Gill get ready to leave, Gary's eyes open. He seems thrilled to see familiar faces. Beverly and Gill promise to return as Gary continues to recuperate. Their visit was really for me and I'm grateful for it. When I get back to the room, I put Beverly's card with Reena's on the right.

The day wears on and I keep flipping though the cards. At 4 p.m. I take my 45-minute power walk around the hall. Beverly's visit energized me and I am practically sprinting. I even pump my arms as I round the floor. As I pass the same rooms over and over again, I wave. I probably look like an idiot.

I grab buffalo chicken salad for dinner and I bring it back to the room. Gary's watching DVD's and eating his chicken dinner.

There are some cooked carrots on the side and applesauce for dessert. Gary is scarfing down this meal. I like this hospital meal. It's not gluten-based and the components are actually in the book. I gently point out that this is the type of food Gary will get to eat on a nutritional plan. He says nothing and takes another bite of chicken. We fall asleep with the "Biggest Loser" blaring on the TV.

I wake up to the usual routine of residents. They seem so sure about what they are doing. I wish I were surer about how to proceed here. This morning Gary is served more flour and sugar for breakfast, pancakes with syrup. Gary devours the stack. Another battle lost.

I start thumbing through the cards again when my cellphone rings. It's Gary Kempinski, one of my best friends. I am sure his card is in the pile that I haven't gone through yet. Now, he is on the phone. Twenty years ago, when he was right out of college, he worked for me as a GE trainee. Today, he is a GE general manager with net income responsibility in the billions of dollars. For the past 20 years, we've spoken weekly on the phone but we rarely meet up in person, even though he lives less than an hour from me. Before he hangs up, he says he's coming to visit this afternoon.

Gary K. is one of the most amazing men I know. When he was new on the job, I was responsible for launching a new consumer business. I needed $5 million of investment from the president of our division. The president said he'd meet with me for 10 minutes and wanted to see a one-page summary of the plan. While it seemed ludicrous to me to summarize all my work on one page, I knew GE: We were efficient. I wanted the funding so bad, my one-pager looked like I was taking an open book science exam and I crammed every fact onto the sheet. I even used six-point font. Gary K. took one look at the sheet. He yelled, "KISS: Keep It Simple, Stupid." He suggested three columns with the titles: Purpose, Process and Payoff. He suggested I should just highlight the major points under each. I got the money within 20 minutes. After that presentation, I knew one day Gary would hold a major leadership position in corporate America. Today, if the business he runs for GE were a separate entity, he would be a very powerful CEO.

Gary looks like the exact corporate mold of a leader. He is 6'2" with a strong build, wavy brown hair, a warm smile and a firm handshake. To me, the most impressive aspect of his personality is that he told me at the age of 23 that he would not suck up to get ahead. His plan was to build the strongest teams and best relationships. In college, he led the Princeton football team to win the Ivy League. As underdogs, it was an incredible victory and a lasting lesson about how to get the most from people.

It is not an accident that my son's name is Gary. When I was pregnant, Steve and I discussed names. In the Jewish heritage it is traditional to name the child after a deceased relative. This is one of the highest honors. When we broke the news to my mom that we planned to name our first son Gary, she said, "You can't do that. Who is he named for?"

"Gary Kempinski," I said.

"That doesn't work!" She screamed it so loud, I thought I felt the baby shudder in my belly.

I looked at her and said nothing. Maybe she realized my mind was made up. "You know," she said, "Uncle Wilbert, your father's brother, his Hebrew name was Gershom. That is like Gary."

I smiled. I knew we'd have to convince my dad and I'd need her help. She continued, "You'll name the baby Gary, after Uncle Wilbert."

It was a stretch, but it worked. Uncle Wilbert would have loved my Gary. They both played tennis and ran cross country.

The day moves at a snail's pace mostly because I am so excited about Gary K.'s arrival this afternoon. I'm stuck wearing the same corduroys that I drag out each day. I select one of my cleaner sweaters. I spend extra time fixing my hair and double-check my makeup, something I'd deny doing if anyone asked me. Besides getting physically ready, I mentally prepare for this visit by going back into corporate mode. Truth be told, I miss the old days. I liked looking good in my suits and having something significant to contribute to meetings. I am so far from that now. Still, I'm spending my morning looking for hospital process improvements. I try to bring a small piece of my professionalism back. I place the laptop on the desk and start writing. After a while, my Gary and I eat lunch, wait for the nurses to shut off the beeping machines and decide to take an afternoon nap. Maybe that will make the day go faster. Gary is also excited about Gary K's visit. They've met a couple of times. My son loves hearing stories about the Princeton football games and about his namesake.

I feel a tap on my shoulder. I open my eyes and it's Gary K. He's earlier than I expected. I wanted to look fresh and fabulous when he came to visit. But after this nap, plus a week in the hospital, and no prep time, I'm afraid I missed that goal. I stand up and I run my fingers through my frizz in an attempt to brush the bushiness down, but know I have the stuck-my-hands-in-a-light-socket electrified hair look going. Naps do that to my hair. Oh well. Gary K. hugs me anyway. As I step back from the embrace, I see my son Gary opening his eyes.

Gary K. walks right over to the bed. He focuses in and says, "How's it going, bud?"

"OK," my son says.

"You've been through so much. I'm so happy to see you," Gary K. says.

After some cursory discussion, I bring up the big decision for my Gary: whether to opt for nutritional therapy when he gets out of here or whether to take the potentially harmful medicines. We haven't had time to discuss it prior to him coming here, but I trust Gary K. enough to help us make the best decision. I go into corporate mode and give a typical corporate elevator speech to briefly review the nutritional route and its requirement to not to eat solid foods for 30 days every three months.

Gary K. knows the job at hand. He looks directly at my son, like I am not even in the room. I just watch as he starts off with, "So, are you thinking about what you can do to keep from coming back here?"

"I know what my mom wants – nutritional therapy – but she doesn't know how hard it is. She can't even fast for one day on Yom Kippur!"

I am wondering if Gary K. even knows what Yom Kippur is.

"Nutritional therapy sounds really hard. Considering all you've been though, you look pretty good. How you feeling now?" Gary K. says.

"Oh, much better. It doesn't hurt to pee!" my son says with pride, almost like he caught the winning touchdown. Gary K. high-fives my son.

"I bet you want to get out of here," Gary K. says.

"Yeah."

I watch in amazement. I know exactly what Gary K. is doing. He is setting the goal. It's why he is such an amazing leader. It's why his teams perform so well. He gets people to focus on the desired result. He gets their buy-in. I sit on the couch and observe a pro in action.

"And never come back," Gary K. says.

I know this is the stretch goal. In GE we always established goals and then even figured out how to surpass the goals. As a GE leader, this came naturally to my friend, Gary K.

"Yeah," my son says again. It is the monosyllable speak that I hate, but at least my son seems engaged.

"So, how can you make that happen?" Gary K. says.

I am watching Gary K. move my child forward. Once the goal is established and agreed upon, a plan is needed. It is business 101, but the challenge is always getting the workforce to execute the plan. I say nothing and act like I am not even in the room.

"I dunno," my son says.

My son is not being disrespectful. He is confused by the question. It's too broad. Even though I believe my son is aware of his options to keep his Crohn's in check – nutritional therapy or medications – he does not connect that he needs to choose a strategy to keep him in remission as long as possible. He looks lost. That vacuous look in his eyes tells me he feels bad at how confused he is. My heart breaks for him. My son is an analytic. He is detail-oriented. He can do steps to a task if he is told what to do but to figure out the game plan, the strategy, that's tough. It's tough even for many grown-ups to figure out a strategy to get a desired result. Many people just start working and hoping it will get them to where they want to be. My son really doesn't know how to proceed. I keep my mouth shut and trust that Gary K. will have the patience to help my son work through the answer. In my years of working with Gary K., I've watched him communicate with people on their level and then help them reach the next level. That's his secret to building consistently winning teams. He builds people up, never tears them down. So, I know he will not belittle my son for not understanding the question. He'll work with him on his level. It's his secret to obtaining unsurpassed loyalty.

"Well it sounds like you have some options for maintaining how good you feel right now," Gary K. tries again.

"Yeah," my son says. I wish Gary would stop with the monosyllables but I just hold my breath and literally sit on my hands. I want to shout out the answer: You have to choose between nutritional therapy or medications! Gary K. knows the options but instead of saying them, he follows the rule: This has to come from the player. This way the person feels some ownership for their idea.

"Tell me about your options," Gary K. directs. There is no question mark at the end of the sentence. The expectation is clear and specific, something within Gary's abilities because it is tactical, it's the details. It's what my son feels comfortable answering.

"Well, I can take some medications. They have side effects. But it's easier than the other choice," my son says with confidence.

"Great, so you have some choices. Tell me about them."

"Well the first is 6-MP. It's a pill. It could affect my liver or pancreas. I don't like that," my son says. I can tell he listened to the doctor.

"I can understand why. What else?" Gary K says.

"Well, there is Remicade. All my friends with Crohn's take it. I'd just go to the hospital every couple of months and they give me an I.V. for a couple of hours. I can eat anything I want." My son says this like it is the best solution. He's not mentioning the part about lymphoma! I keep my mouth shut. Gary K. has had lots of experience with people trying to convince him to invest in big projects and how it can look rosy at first glance. Gary K. knows how to probe. But, in order not to shut the other person down when questioning he needs to seem supportive. So, I am not surprised with his response. "That sounds real good. Any negatives?"

"Teenage boys have a higher chance of lymphoma," my son admits.

Without judgment, Gary K. goes for clarification, "Oh, lymphoma, that's cancer right?" (How can you not love this guy?)

"Yeah."

"Other options?" Gary K. asks.

"Nutritional therapy."

"What is that?"

My son responds, "Well, I can eat anything I want for three months and then the next month I only drink a supplement. They said they can teach me to put a tube up my nose into my stomach so I can feed myself during my sleep."

"So, you have three choices. Nice," Gary K. says.

"Yeah."

"So, all three will help keep you in remission," Gary K. says.

"Yeah."

"Well, did your Mom ever tell you about a QFD?" Gary K. says.

Of course I did! I think this but I don't say it.

"Yeah, we use it a lot. She showed it to me when I had to choose between French or Spanish in middle school. It helped me pick the best choice for me," my son says. Ah, Gary. You do listen to me! My son is so excited that he knows this GE tool that he starts telling Gary K. how it works. "I list my goals on the left side of the page and then I put my options along the top. Then I rank each option on a scale of one to five, based on meeting the goal on the left. My mom taught me to put it in Excel so it automatically adds up the numbers. The one with the highest score wins."

Said like a pro. I look at Gary K. and he smiles. Adults struggle with making decisions every day. It's hard when there are many reasons why each choice might be the best. How do you quantify the options to make the best decision? I am beaming because clearly my son learned how to make decisions using this advanced Six Sigma quality tool. The QFD or Quantitative Functional Deployment, is a big phrase that means how do you find a numeric way to quantify what is the best deployment of a function? Simply, it's a strategic tool used by corporations to get employees to make the best choice when there are so many options available. The whole point is to take the emotion out of it.

"Well it could work for you here as well," Gary K. states. "You say your goals are to stay out of the hospital and stay healthy." He looks at my son and adds "Actually, do you really think we need to do a QFD for this?"

"No," my son says.

"Why not?"

"Because the Remicade might put me back here with a disease that could kill me. So that choice is out. The other choice might hurt my liver. No way will that score high," my son says.

My son looks up at Gary K., who looks fit and trim. My son finally says, "Just that I hate not eating."

"I bet," Gary K. says.

"It's really hard," my son says, verging on tears. My heart is breaking for him. He's right. I could never do it.

"You've done nutritional therapy before and what were the side effects?" Gary K. says.

"Boredom."

"So, couldn't you try it and keep the other options as back-up plans. You'll know they are there for you if you need them," Gary K. says.

"Yeah. I can try this. I don't have to stay with it. Maybe it won't be so tough," my son says, trying to convince himself.

"Gary, I think you can do this. You are amazing. You've already done it," Gary K. says.

My son turns to me and asks, "Mom, can I go to Sakura before I start and after I end each time?"

I shout out, "Yeah!" The perfect one syllable response.

And just like that, my son Gary decides to implement nutritional therapy.

"Keep me posted on your progress. I believe in you!" Gary K. says as he walks toward the door.

I walk him to the elevator. We don't say much to each other. We don't have to. As I walk back to the room, I wish Big Gary or someone could teach the doctors how to help patients make choices. Protocol bombards patients with information but not the skills to narrow down the key parameters and choose wisely.

I sit down on the couch and watch Gary eat a hamburger for dinner. He tells me he is going to skip the bun because he is watching his gluten. The phone rings and I am so happy I sound like I am singing hello. It is my friend Julie. She asks how Gary is doing. I tell her he's just decided he will not eat solid food for a month at a time for the rest of his life. She listens and after about five minutes, she is talking about her career and whether she'll be able to retire in five years. It's a replay of how she handled my car accident so I am not surprised this time by her choice of conversation. Instead of ending the friendship, I am clear with my needs. In the same firm tone Gary K. used with my son, I say, "Julie thanks for calling. When Gary is well, we can talk about this. I'll call you soon."

She breaks in not wanting me to hang up. "What can I do?" she says.

After 20 years of friendship, I accept she is a detail-oriented person. She needs help with the big picture. She wants to be on the team. She just needs to be led. "Send flowers and a card," I suggest.

The next day her card and a huge beautiful floral arrangement and balloons arrive saying, "Get well soon." I place the flowers on the windowsill and their fragrance fills the room. I put her card on the right. Gary and I go to sleep at night and it smells like spring.

What You Can Do Now

---

1. Get to know other parents in the hospital.

Listen to their stories. This might help you gain perspective about how to deal with your current situation.

2. Accept the limitations of your friends/family.

Many will say the wrong thing. It is not their fault. Most probably they have not experienced what you are going through. Instead of correcting them, just say you'll speak to them when things improve. Figure out which of your friends/family members can be most supportive. Be selective. Quality beats quantity in this case. Let them know you are counting on them. Ask if they can be especially supportive during this time. Don't assume they have capacity for you.

3. Master the QFD. (visit www.RandiRedmondOster.com/QFD)

To figure out the best option, when you have to make a difficult decision, make a chart. On the left, list your goals. Give the goal a weight, with one being low; three, medium; and five, high. In columns across the top of the page, write the options you can pursue to achieve the goal. For each option, score how well the option meets the goal. Use the same scoring (one/low, three/medium, five/high). Multiply the weight times the score and enter the product in the box. Total the numbers vertically. The highest score is the best option. If two are close, you can choose one to implement.

Goals	Weight	Option 1	Option 2	Option 3	Option 4
TOTAL					

Chapter 10
Hello, Miss Connecticut;
Goodbye, Dr. Freud

I hear the tiptoes of residents approaching. Apparently they're heeding my requests for a softer wake-up. They no longer turn on the lights and descend in unison speaking at the top of their lungs for their morning rounds, at least not with Gary. And more and more nurses are replacing Gary's I.V. bags before the machine beeps. I think the fact that I am writing about my experiences in the hospital has helped some staff become more aware of their practices. Just seeing Gary being handled gently in a soft lit room is making the day start better. For this I am grateful.

Today, one resident brought in a flashlight. I noticed the beam on the desk. Maybe the resident was trying to check out the feedback sheet, the one with the names of people I will be including in a thank-you letter to the hospital CEO. I've noticed more and more people trying to sneak a peek at the list as they walk in the room. It's difficult to do this discretely in the dark, though.

After the residents leave, a nursing manager brings in a student nurse. I've never seen this student before. The nurse manager glances at the list before she approaches Gary. (She's already made the list.) The blonde student with dimples looks slightly older than Gary. The nurse manager tells her to press this, remove that, watch for air pockets here. I sense that the student's tentative movements with the equipment means she is green. Now, the nurse manager wants her to insert an I.V. into Gary. The manager tells me this will be Molly's first time inserting the I.V. on a real patient. She asks my permission and I turn to Gary – it's his arm after all. Gary smiles at her, probably because he thinks she's cute. He tells her about the list and lets her know that if she does it well, we'll add her name. I hope this doesn't make her more nervous! The student nurse takes Gary's forearm. She shakes as she brings the needle close to his arm. I hold my breath. She stabs him but no blood comes out. The manager encourages her to try again. Her hand shakes even more. Gary doesn't move an inch. He winces but he doesn't make a sound. The I.V. goes in. All he says once it's in is, "You did great. Mom, add Molly to the list!"

Molly is beaming. Her manager gives me a wink as they leave.

Later, as usual, I take out my laptop and record the interaction. As I am typing away, Dr. Simmon enters the room to check on Gary. He glances at the list on the counter but says nothing. He's still not on there. As he walks over to Gary he appears uneasy. I smile as I look up from the laptop, to see if that changes his demeanor. Before he even says hello to Gary, he asks me, "You get to the plane part yet?" Our brief conversation with him in the plane on the runway seems to be foremost in his mind.

I smile and say, "Not yet. But remember it is only part of a whole story. We still have to see this through to a beautiful ending."

"Let's see if we can turn around how I come across," he says, sincerely.

I like Dr. Simmon. I like that he is direct and concerned about how he handled communicating with me during his absence. But my goal isn't about my likes or dislikes. It's about trying to get the best care for my son. He walks over to Gary and smiles. He recites the protocol questions about gas, eating and defecating. He asks to look at Gary's belly. When the doctor presses down I don't hear Gary yelp. Wow, that's a good sign! Plus, I notice the redness has not traveled outside the line. He tells Gary how wonderful everything looks and he goes and sits on the couch. That's a first. I suspect he is here for a conversation about next steps. I sit in the chair next to

Gary's bed.

Dr. Simmon asks, "Have you thought about keeping your Crohn's in remission?"

Gary blurts out, "I've made my decision."

I am thrilled to see Gary take ownership.

"Really, what are you thinking?" Dr. Simmon asks.

"Nutritional therapy," Gary proclaims. I feel total relief.

"Great choice, if you can do it. Many teenagers don't even have this option and many of those that do, can't do it. But, Gary, you can. You've done it before," he says. That's the spirit, Dr. Simmon!

"When you get out of here, you'll eat food for the first month. I'll set up a training session with a nurse and she'll teach you how to insert the NG tube yourself at home. It's a much smaller tube than the one in the hospital. I have one other boy doing it and he says he doesn't even feel it," Dr. Simmon says.

"Great," says Gary. "I can eat anything?"

"Well, stay away from seeds, popcorn. But that is about it."

Unbelievable. He's not even acknowledging a connection between Crohn's and diet – except for the food that can get stuck. His idea of nutritional therapy is to eat as you like, but to just give your intestines a month-break by only drinking liquids a couple of times a year. I understand resting the intestines. I figure the digestive track is like the internal plumbing of the body. The large and small intestines are the pipes. The same way excessive Drano usage can hurt pipes, I guess some foods are as caustic.

But Dr. Simmon doesn't mention anything about good and bad bacteria. He doesn't even mention eating yogurt, which has natural probiotics that the good bacteria love and that keep the intestines performing at their peak. I've read that good bacteria can help reduce inflammation. I bet there are foods besides seeds that are an irritant to the intestine. How about gluten? What about high fructose corn syrup? What about Gary's favorite breakfast – French toast from white bread with artificial maple syrup?

I think all this, but I don't say a word. Besides, the doctor already told me Gary isn't gluten intolerant, so I shouldn't even worry about that. Maybe French toast isn't so bad. I'll just buy pure maple syrup. And make it on whole wheat bread. I keep my mouth shut. With a firm handshake, Dr. Simmon leaves.

I love to eat. For me, Gary's challenge of not eating solid food for a month would be even greater than designing the entire electronic combat system of the Stealth Fighter. I know: My team did it. Now, Gary believes he can do this. He can follow a wise path to healing.

Gary is glowing. He looks so happy with his decision. It seems that a weight has been lifted off of him – and me. I pull out my laptop to continue the journal and record this milestone.

It's rare, but Gary interrupts my typing and starts talking.

"Mom, you know it's weird here."

I look up from the keyboard. "In what way?"

"My dreams are so intense," he says.

"Really?" I've noticed the same thing with my dreams! They say medications and anesthesia can make dreams much more vivid but I am experiencing the same thing and I am not on anything.

"Yeah. Like last night I had a dream. Normally, I don't remember them. But this…"

"What did you dream?"

"It was about the whole family. We had to escape through this little hole in a wall. To get out we had to climb up and squeeze through. Matt did it easily. Even you did. Dad struggled because it was so small. I was so scared he'd get stuck."

"What happened?"

"You pulled him and I pushed him. He made it," Gary says.

"What about you?"

"At first I couldn't reach the hole in the wall. It was so hard. Everyone else was on the other side. I struggled and struggled. I was so pissed. I almost gave up. But I finally reached the hole. Then you guys helped me through."

I am not a dream expert but this seems obvious to me. Subconsciously, he knows he can get through the wall. But, I say nothing. It has to click for him. Gary has to link the dream to his life. I want to talk so bad, but that will take away this teachable moment in which he can teach himself. So, I start to count silently to myself, to the number eight. I know in general people hate awkward silence and will break it by the time I hit that magic number. It works almost every time! I smile and start counting. One, two, three, four ... still he says nothing. I want to talk so bad. Five, six...

Gary blurts out, "Know what? I know what that dream means. I'm going to make it!"

I put down the laptop and give him a hug. I am grateful for his belief in himself. I know this is the most important element for his success. I've led many teams at work that were supposedly comprised of the "C" players, the underperformers. Over time they became high-performing teams. The key was that each person took ownership of his or her job. I couldn't do their work for them. I could tell them they were capable, but they had to believe it. I see that Gary believes in himself, and that's the greatest asset a person can possess. Often, it's the only way a person can handle high pressure and still perform.

I hear a knock on the door. It is Dr. Arnold, Gary's psychotherapist, the one the E.R. required him to see back when they kept saying his seizure-like episodes were from anxiety. After the endocrinologist discovered that Gary was hypoglycemic, Gary never had an attack again. But he kept going to the therapist each week. I'd try to listen through the door to hear what they were talking about. Does he really have anxiety? Is he telling the doctor I am a bad mother? I never went to a therapist, so I'm not sure what they do. I know many people are helped by them, but I am afraid to be analyzed. The only reason I didn't cancel the appointments was because Gary told me he liked talking to Dr. Arnold. Since the sessions are only partially covered by insurance, Steve and I doled out the hundreds of dollars a month. However, unlike our rabbi, who has never visited the hospital, I'm impressed that Dr. Arnold makes the hour-and-a-half trek to see Gary.

I size up Dr. Arnold and he seems uneasy. He is a man in his 50's and looks like the kind of guy a casting director would hire to play a therapist role – gray hair, slightly paunchy, wearing wire-rimmed glasses. His brow is furrowed with wrinkles. I'm guessing he doesn't like hospitals. I don't know him well, except for mostly discussing the bills – and my attempts at eavesdropping – but maybe hospitals are a personal issue for him. I've been here so long, I am becoming more and more at ease in the environment and I suspect so is Gary. Dr. Arnold requests to talk privately with Gary. I am not surprised; it's what they always do. Gary seems happy to see him. They shoo me out of the room.

I use the 50-minute hour for my power walk. When I return I am slightly sweaty but knock on Gary's room's door. Gary is beaming. I'll never know what they talked about but Dr. Arnold asks to speak to me privately as well. We stand in the hall. After all, it's too complicated to get Gary out of the room with all the equipment he is hooked up to. I don't want to be analyzed. I am uncomfortable talking with the therapist. I don't want to just start blurting out stuff. I lean against the wall and start counting to eight. Dr. Arnold leans up against the wall in the same position. Aha – he's using the mirroring technique, which I used in sales to get my prospects more comfortable with me. But this makes me feel even more uneasy! The silence is killing me. I get to the number seven and blurt out, "How's Gary seem to you?"

Dr. Arnold tells me that one reason he'd felt Gary had anxiety was because Dr. Arnold felt that Gary wasn't telling him his real feelings. He refers to a time Gary defecated in the woods during a high school cross country practice. The kids run five miles around town. Gary had to go to the bathroom. There was no place to go. So, Gary told the other kids to go on while he did his business. Gary told

Dr. Arnold the story and that it was not a big deal. I believed Gary, but Dr. Arnold had told me this is a very embarrassing situation, especially for teenagers. He used some therapist lingo to explain this is traumatic, something about bodily functions and Freud. I don't know. I never studied this stuff. To Dr. Arnold, Gary clearly was not dealing with his feelings. I know Gary is used to defecating in the woods. We go hiking frequently and you "go" when you need to go. I've never made a big deal of pooping in the woods. You go, you clean up after yourself and you move on. I guess I've taught him it's a normal bodily function. To me, I can't believe my ears. I am paying all of this money because Gary is telling him the truth, but the textbook says Gary should feel traumatized. What do I know? Now, Dr. Arnold looks me in the eye and says, "I don't think he has anxiety. I think those seizures were a complication of the Crohn's."

Thank you and goodbye, Dr. Freud.

We've been here two Wednesdays now. Wednesday is pet therapy day. We carefully move the tubing from the pumping machine to make room for the dog. A golden retriever jumps up on Gary's bed and lies down next to Gary, who lights up as he pets the dog. I am so amazed at how well trained the dog is. We're impressed when our family dog, Chloe, follows the "sit" command. She could never handle this job.

It's Halloween and the hospital staff really tries to make the day special. Instead of the kids getting dressed up to go trick-or-treating, the nurses and even some special visitors dress up and bring the candy and small trinkets to the kids. Miss Connecticut even comes to the hospital! She dresses up as a witch and cavorts with the press. They take her picture as she prances around the floor. She enters Gary's room and I guess it's her PR manager who asks Gary if he'd like to take a picture with the most beautiful girl in the state. Gary doesn't seem impressed but he nods yes to be polite and she walks over and gives him a kiss as he lies in the bed with the tubes. Later he doesn't even post the picture on Facebook. He's tired of this place. I think he'd rather have his grandma kiss him then have to hang out in the hospital with the beauty queen. Would Dr. Arnold find this strange as well? The day drags on.

The next day, we both wake up wanting out. Why is it that the closer you are to the destination the longer it seems to take to get there? Every second drags on. There is not a dog, a clown, a beautiful girl that can get Gary to want to spend another minute here waiting around to see what other entertainment will arrive. This morning Gary is no longer hooked up to machines. The nurses followed doctors' orders and removed them. He can walk freely around the entire floor, albeit slowly. He says he still has incision pain, but none from his insides. He tells me he can tell the difference between pains and once he heals he's going to be great. The only thing keeping Gary from hospital dismissal is one poop. It is his ticket to leave. This morning during rounds, the residents said they could feel and hear Gary's system working. There is a poop in there. It is just a matter of time for it to be released.

The protocol train no longer seems like an enigma to me. It is predictable and, with the tweaked patient relations, Gary and I are much more comfortable. Now, the residents are consistently quiet in the morning. The nurses over-communicate what they are doing and why. The doctors keep touching Gary's belly and listening through the stethoscope. They keep reassuring us that everything looks and sounds good. They, too, over-communicate with us.

Dr. Simmon says recovery is typically three weeks. Gary will be able to go home and start practicing for the tennis team in December. Gary is excited because he believes this will give him enough time to be ready for March tryouts. What excites me the most is to see Gary's determination. He keeps asking me to arrange a couple of private lessons with his tennis coach so he can catch up. I don't wait till the count of eight to say yes.

"I am leaving today, Mom," Gary says as a statement, not a question.

"We have to wait for the poop," I say.

"I am leaving today. Pack my bags. I am ready to go. I am standing here by the door," he says, sounding like John Denver in the old top-40 tune "I'm Leaving on a Jet Plane."

I decide not to tell him the refrain to the song mentions not knowing when he'll be back again.

As I type about the day's activity, Gary's surgeon comes in around 11 a.m. to assess Gary's progress. Gary insists that the doctor release him today. Gary refuses to take no for an answer. He doesn't want to wait around to poop. He tells the doctor he'll do it at home. I love his conviction. I let him lead this one. Finally, the doctor agrees to sign the discharge paperwork. The doctor explains that it needs to be processed and then we will be free to leave. Gary high-fives the doctor before he walks toward the door.

I become a busy bee. I get a red wagon from the nurses' station and place several of the stuffed animals and flowers in it and take it to the car. The rest I give to the nurses to give to other children on the floor. I move the car to the valet parking so it will be easy for Gary to exit later. I pack the bags. I clean the room. I move so quickly that everything is done in one hour. The room looks like the sterile, cold place it was on the first day we arrived. Gary puts on his own clothes for the first time in 15 days. He looks great. We just sit on the edge of his bed and wait and wait for the paperwork. I don't think time can move any slower. I put my laptop in the car. I have nothing to do. Sitting idly is definitely not my strength.

Finally, there is a knock on the door. I glance at my watch. It's 3:30 p.m. A nurse tells us they have the final signature. We can go. She asks Gary to sit in the wheelchair. An attendant wheels Gary into the elevator. We go down to the first floor and I hand my name sticker to the guard. Every day, I had to put it on my sweater so I could roam about the hospital corridors freely. It's so used up, it barely sticks to my sweater. I got my mileage off that ticket. I see the new crop of passengers entering. The newbies' stickers are white and fresh. Their adventure is about to begin. I can only hope their outcome is as good as Gary's.

Gary gets up from the wheelchair and chooses to walk out the door, holding his head high. I follow right behind him. It's a cold crisp fall day with the orange sun hanging low in the sky. Gary takes a slow step outside. I see him take a deep breath and release, the kind of deep breath that would score a 1,000 on the breathing machine. Gary inhales the fresh air like it is a gift.

The valet brings us the car and the hour-and-a-half drive home is full of Gary discussing catching up in school, getting ready for tennis tryouts and playing with Chloe. He sounds like he is in over-drive. I wish Steve could see this but he is still in New Jersey. He should be home tomorrow night. As I pull into the garage, I hear Chloe bark like crazy, so much more than usual. It's like she can tell Gary is with me. Gary takes the cane and walks slowly into the kitchen. Chloe jumps up on him. Grandma screams at the dog: "You'll destroy the stitches. Get out of here!" Matthew runs for a dog treat to lure Chloe into the basement.

I am home.

I smell Chinese food and see our neighbors, Keith Buckman and his son Mitch, sitting at the table. They are the first to bear meals. Gary loves Chinese food and I am so grateful I don't have to cook. Gary invites Keith and his son to join us. Sitting at the table with Matt, Grandma, Gary and our friends makes this the best Chinese food ever. It's not long afterward we finally fall asleep in our own beds in our own home. If only Steve could be next to me.

In the morning I hear Gary exclaim, "It still doesn't hurt to pee!" I look out the window and the bright sunshine reflects exactly how I am feeling. There are no residents here to wake me up. My butt didn't slip between the cracks of couch cushions. I feel like I could just stand next to the ice-covered walkway and it would melt. Gary ambles over to me with his cane. His stride is slower than Grandma's. He doesn't complain of any surgery pain.

"You know, Mom, it feels great to just be able to get up in the morning and go to the bathroom, without having to wait 30 minutes for the pain to go away. I feel great."

As good as that sounds, I am a bit nervous. I pulled him out of the hospital before the "big" event. "Any poop yet?"

"Nope," he says like who the hell cares. He is so happy. Then he adds, "I bet most people take for granted just getting up in the morning without pain. Today is a great day."

Gary holds his side with one hand and the cane with the other. Each step seems to hurt. He slowly walks toward the top of the stairs. I grab my glasses and follow him. Gary looks at the stairs like they are a downward ski slope packed with ice: treacherous. I just want him well and it pains me to see him struggle with such simple things like stairs. He's gone backward in physical development and needs me more than ever for basic things, like dressing and grabbing his clothes from the closet. This is going to be a long haul for him … and me. He doesn't seem frustrated, though, because he truly believes he will get better. I shut my mouth because it looks like to me he is being overly cautious. I think of all the things an impatient parent could say, like "C'mon, it's only stairs" or "Stop acting like this is worse than the surgery." But I don't say a word. I am not sure how to not baby him while getting him to man up.

Seeing him struggle makes me wonder if he'll be ready for tennis tryouts in March. The doctor says he can start practicing mid December. But, looking at him on these stairs, I doubt he'll progress fast enough. Now that we're home, I don't have the patience for this. My New York roots creep up. I want it fast, now. I shut my mouth and will him down the steps.

"Hey, Gary, you got down faster than you got up the stairs last night. Nice," I say. I hope he doesn't detect the artificial sweetener in my tone.

"Mom, can you make me eggs for breakfast?"

"Sure, with your help. You are the best scrambler. I'll be down in a few."

I take a long hot shower. The big bar of oatmeal lavender soap is my favorite. I inhale its smell. As the hot water washes away the hospital germs, I stop feeling guilty for not rushing downstairs to whip up Gary's eggs and Matt's favorite breakfast of waffles. It's been weeks since I've spent real time with Matt. I'll make his favorite lunch today. Right now, the water pressure is perfect for rinsing my hair. Now, I can finally shave my legs and underarms.

I dry off and wrap a big, fluffy bath towel around my body. They didn't have those in the hospital. I hear my mom, Gary and Matt laughing downstairs. I walk over to the top of the stairs. I think I smell French toast. Matt loves Grandma's French toast.

Grandma screams so the whole world can hear, "I am not the slowest anymore. Look, I can even get up out of my chair faster than Gary!"

I hear Matt say, "You guys race. Who can get up out of the chair first? Get on your mark, get set … Go."

I tuck the towel around me and run downstairs. I've got to see this. Gary bursts out laughing as he struggles to stand up. I am laughing right along with them. Grandma uses her cane for balance, stands up and wins.

"You cheated. You used your cane," Gary jokes.

"Ah, next time you'll use yours," Grandma says, knowing she can teach him a thing or two.

My mom is using the same technique she used to raise me. It is as if I can see the thoughts in her head: Work with what you have. Accept your obstacles and find a way to overcome them. Don't make excuses. Laugh instead of complain. I feel so blessed she lives with us. She is going to help me make Gary's progress fun. I'm going to race the two of them until he wins.

Matt tells me he has to work today. He takes care of our neighbors' three cats whenever Seth and Laurie go on vacation. The cats are outdoor and indoor wanderers. Whiskers is a white and brown, long-haired, overweight cat and is special to our family. In the spring and summer, he comes by our pond to catch a frog for dinner. He is a great hunter and I think he even taught other neighborhood cats the skill. Matt and I love to sit on the deck and watch Whiskers sit on a boulder beside the pond, just waiting for the perfect time to pounce. It can take hours. Matt seems to have the same patience level because he'll sit and wait and just watch until Whiskers finds his next meal. Not me, I'm too busy racing to my next thing and screaming out, "Did he get it yet?"

My mom describes Matt as the type of kid that her grandma, from Russia, sent at age 12 to the United States before WWI. Great-Uncle Mac found a job while he was an adolescent and sent money back for the rest of the family to make the trip. I know my mother is not exaggerating because Matt started an animal care business at nine and in the last three years it's grown to seven clients. He takes care of everything from horses, dogs, fish, birds and plants. Sometimes before school he has to get up super early to feed four horses and five cats. Matt is trusted with all of our neighbors' keys. I know my mom is right about him. If I had to, I'd send him to the New World confident he would thrive.

I think that helps me feel less guilt about not being there for him.

Matt bundles up and leaves. I just assume he'll put on boots, gloves and a hat. While I watch Gary take every slow step to the bathroom to see if he'll poop already, I stay outside the door. I hear Gary gleefully exclaim, "I feel it coming."

It's been over an hour of Gary telling me it's almost here. I think Whiskers catches a frog faster than this poop is coming. I start to notice that Matt is not back yet and wonder if he is OK. But each time I want to leave to find Matt, Gary says, "I feel it." I can tell he wants me there for the victory flush! I hate feeling so torn between the two and picking one over the other. As I stand outside the bathroom door, I think about Cathy and how she must feel with one who is autistic and the other, paraplegic. Whom do you pay attention to? Just thinking of Cathy makes me put my situation in perspective. My mom's uncle survived in steerage on a ship as he crossed the Atlantic; Matt can handle a short trek in the snow to the neighbors' house.

After another 30 minutes of waiting and waiting, I am about to get my coat and leave. Gary screams, "Come in and take a look. I did it!"

My mom and I go in the bathroom. It's a gas factory in here. I hold my nose, my mom starts gagging. Yet, she still takes her cane to inch closer to the toilet to see it. I peer in as well. Gary's system is working! We high-five each other as Matt comes in, looking dejected. He doesn't even comment about the smell.

"Gary pooped!" I exclaim. I know I am making it a big deal and probably too big of a deal considering Matt has given Grandma her eye drops every night, has done all of this homework and has straight A's in school.

"Great," Matt says with a matter-of-fact tone. It is not typical of him to be disinterested, and especially not when such big news just happened.

I say to him, "What's up?"

"Mom, Whiskers is sleeping and won't get up. Can you come see him?"

I tell Gary to call the doctor with his news then I bundle up and walk through the snow to our neighbors' house. Their house is a country cottage on three acres, surrounded by tall pines with bird feeders in the backyard and a cat door on a screen porch for the strays. There are no sidewalks between our houses and the snow is much higher than I thought, taller than my boots. My socks are soaked and my feet melt the snow. I feel frozen as Matt opens the side door.

It's rare for me to be in my neighbors' house. I can see they clearly love their cats. There is cat fur on the furniture, lots of worn-out stuffed animal play toys and a slight cat smell in the house. I bet it's not noticeable to them. Matt points me downstairs to the finished basement. I see Whiskers lying at the bottom of the stairs. I pet him. He is cold to the touch. He is stiff.

He is dead.

A couple of feet away it looks like he exploded diarrhea before he died. The smell is worse than what I just left with Gary. I start to gag. I never had time to eat breakfast so I just dry heave.

"Are you OK, Mom? Is Whiskers going to be OK?" Matt whispers from up the stairs.

I see Matt looking like the boy he really is, not the man I keep telling myself is ready for the New World. I come up and I put my arm around him and whisper, "Whiskers died, honey."

"I thought so, Mom. He's stiff." Matt wells up.

Maybe other parents would try to soften the blow. Maybe it's a mistake that I've always dealt directly with my kids. Like with the tooth fairy. I clearly told them when they were five, I was the tooth fairy. They still got the crisp dollar bill, but there was no innocence about the mystery of who placed it there. I tell him Whiskers will always be in our hearts and I hug him tightly.

"Let's make a casket for him so when they come back they can bury him," I suggest.

"OK, dust to dust," Matt says. He seems comforted by knowing the circle of life and doesn't ask me if the cat is in heaven.

"Before we make the casket, we have to clean up the poop," I say. "Can you get me some paper towels?"

Matt says the smell is too bad for him and he'd rather be in charge of the casket. So, I send him home to find a box. It is the least I can do for him. I clean up my neighbors' cat poop on the oriental rug after I've spent the last week waiting every day for Gary to poop. I can't help but think of the elephants flying around my head and pooping right now. I actually smirk in between gags because I know the secret, clean up one at a time. I place the paper towels in a plastic bag and spray some Lysol on the rug. For some reason the morning is all about shit, but I feel like I am doing exactly what I should be doing. I'm not an executive anymore, but my kids need me and my neighbors need me. I imagine the elephants dancing around my head and I scream, "Bring it on!"

I trek back home and Matt has a cardboard box the size of a small toaster on the kitchen table and a bunch of crayons, glue and paper. We decorate the box together. He writes in big letters – "Whiskers: BEST CAT EVER!" It's the first art project we've done in a long time. Granted it's a cat casket, but he seems thrilled to have my attention. We put red hearts on the box and he finds some blue glue with silver glitter and squeezes out the bottle over the letters BEST CAT EVER. You can't miss how special he feels this cat is. In the past, I probably would have been more practical and annoyed with him using the slow-drying glue: It's so messy. It takes too much time. Instead, I just enjoy watching him decorate the box. I snap a mental picture for my moment memory.

"It's done, Mom. Let's go put him in it."

We bundle up again. Matt carries our homemade casket over the snow, careful not to ruin the wet glitter glue. I go downstairs with the decorated box and place it next to Whiskers. I notice the glue is not near dry and some glitter is on my hand. I pick up the stiff cat. It is my first time handling something dead. I hate touching it. I try to place Whiskers in the box, but he doesn't fit. I don't want the box to fall over because it'll ruin the rug. I can't let the cat brush the side of the box because he'll look like we dressed him in a Mardi Gras mask. I try lowering him one more time into the box. I try folding his legs underneath his torso so he'll fit. Nothing budges because the cat is stiffer than a board. Matt yells down suggestions, like move his head, stick his feet up. The more I maneuver the animal the more sparkly the cat and I get and the more Matt laughs, probably a nervous laughter. But I'm glad he sees the humor in our spending an hour decorating the box and now trying to squish the dead cat inside. The silver glitter glue is now on my face, my coat, the cat and our neighbors' rug. I burst out laughing as well. I can't believe I feel happy in the mess and holding a dead cat. Is this my new perspective?

"Matt, let's go home and find another box," I suggest.

This time, Matt finds a very large computer box. We decorate it with even bigger letters and more glitter glue. It's like a cat mausoleum! No one will ever doubt Whiskers is the BEST CAT EVER. The box is so big we put bags of ice in it to keep the cat cold for the next couple of days until Seth and Laurie's return. Luckily, it's almost winter and they have a screened-in porch where we place Whiskers. Matt places the box facing the door so when they come home, they will see "BEST CAT EVER" in shining silver glue. Matt and I kiss the mausoleum and say a prayer. I hold Matt's hand. We walk together back to our house. Whiskers' death feels like the end of an era. We met him the first day we moved in. Now I feel a new beginning, an even brighter one, because I am learning to make something positive out of so much shit.

I open the door as Gary yells from upstairs, "Let's go to Wild Rice for lunch, Mom." It's the same thing he said after the PSATs only 10 weeks ago, but it seems like a lifetime ago. I run upstairs to wash up and put on a little blush and mascara. I look in the mirror and notice a couple of new gray hairs framing some new worry lines. I've earned the right to look my age! The thought of Gary eating his favorite meal at his favorite restaurant covers up any concerns I have about an aging face.

"We'll all go. Grandma, get your cane," I yell upstairs, "we are going to lunch."

"I'll be down as fast as I can. Tell Gary to bring his cane too. He's going to see how he'll need it."

What You Can Do Now

---

1. Give feedback.

If you want your child not to be disturbed when sleeping, tell the nurses and residents your expectations. I found when I was clear with expectations they were reasonable people and wanted to accommodate us.

2. Count to eight.

Instead of talking first, count to eight in your head. Most people will break the silence by then. I found when I let Gary verbalize what was happening to him, he got the point more easily. By listening instead of talking, I got to hear the patient's point of view without force-feeding him mine.

3. Add another dose of patience during recovery.

Recovery takes time. Appreciate daily progress instead of fixating on how far there still is to go.

* * *

Chapter 11
Gary vs. Grandma

Day One of home recovery continues. We're going to use Grandma as a barometer to measure Gary's pace. She struggles every day with crippling arthritis pain and chooses not to complain about it. She challenges, "Let's see how many days it takes you to beat me down the stairs." She is slow and steady. In round one, Grandma beats Gary down the stairs. She tells him how to hold on to the railing and the wall for balance. She bursts out laughing because someone in the house finally understands life from her perspective. Based on how Gary is moving, she'll probably be in the lead for at least a week. I'm sure she'll love not being the last one to the car, getting in the car and getting out of the car. I always have to calculate this extra time when I need to get someplace on time.

Now, I have two trying their best not to be last.

The waiter at Wild Rice seems genuinely excited to see us. We've been away a lot longer than usual. He knows Gary's regular dish and now he has two Jewish mothers reminding him, "NO SEEDS!" Seeds are among the few things even Dr. Simmon says to avoid. Their hard little shells can get jammed in Gary's intestines. I think I say this out loud with my mom and repeat it so many times that Gary is totally embarrassed to be with us. I ask Gary to show his scars to the waiter. He complies, I think to show off a little and to shut me up.

When the food arrives I inspect it for seeds. I am a neurotic mom again and will not let Gary eat a bite until I approve. My mom joins in the seed scrutiny. Gary snatches a California roll with the chopsticks and yells, "Enough already! It's like a stereo with you two." Gary tells the waiter he is living in a Seinfeld episode and that this one should be called "The Seed." America, he said, would crack up with the retort, "No seeds for you!"

The owner of the restaurant, hearing our commotion, comes over and reassures us that there are NO SEEDS. He says in his accent, "You special customers. We not use seeds ever, OK?"

All the quiet customers (in other words, everyone but us) are trying very hard to be polite but are in fact staring at us. Gary picks up another piece of California roll and holds it aloft with his chopsticks for the entire restaurant to see. "No seeds, so I can eat it." We are making a total scene, with our Bronx best trumping our Connecticut etiquette. "I just got out of the hospital," Gary explains to the onlookers, "and this is my first meal out."

After lunch the race to leave is on! After the seed episode, Gary does not seem to care that people see him struggle more than his grandma to get up out of the chair. I don't think he can be any more embarrassed by us. The waiter hands them their respective canes and Matt yells out, "Get on your mark. Get set. Go!"

Customers shout from their tables and everyone in the restaurant seems to root for Gary, the underdog. He tries to walk as fast as Grandma to the exit, but she wins. She takes a bow. The place erupts with applause. I remember again why I love Fairfield. Grandma gloats on the sidewalk, then makes her way to the car.

"Catch me, catch me," she teases.

"I'm trying," Gary yells in between laughs. They look like they're both in pain but all they're doing is laughing, not complaining. I take a mental picture. They're in front of a large window storefront of a business called "Home and Companions," a business that provides homecare for the elderly. Several employees sit at their desks and watch Gary and Grandma "race." I roll my eyes and shake my head at one woman inside who looks like a 40-ish home health care aide. She gives me the thumbs-up sign, which I take to mean that I'm doing a good job sandwiched between elder care and child care.

We finally get to the car and I want to keep everyone moving. Grandma has been bugging me to get a new dishtowel, because ours is apparently too tattered. (I've not been home to notice.) I decide to drive this motley crew to Kohl's. To me, the $3 dishtowel, which she says is imperative to get, NOW, is worth getting NOW if it means she and Gary will get exercise by hobbling through the store. The shopping cart is the best walker ever. Its wheels let customers zip steadily along. Gary and Grandma won't need their canes once they get the carts.

We enter the store to search for shopping carts and three teenage girls whiz pass Grandma. She seems unsteady on her cane and in the nick of time Matt maneuvers a cart into her hands. She regains her composure. Gary just stares at the girls in their too short skirts and belly-button-baring fitted sweaters, his eyes wandering from their Ugg boots over leggings until he stops at their V-necks. I don't think he finishes to their faces. They hold up different skimpy shirts, deciding which color to buy. They glance at Gary, holding onto his cane and quickly return to scrutinizing the shirts. I can't tell how he feels by their reaction – or rather by their complete lack of one. They ignore him. I admit from my own experience that when I see someone with a disability I ignore them because I don't know what I'm supposed to do. I make them invisible while I go about my day. It's like if I don't acknowledge them, their problems won't interfere with my life. My mom says it's not just the disabled who are ignored. She says women become invisible to men and even other woman as they age. I don't dwell on this and I stick to my plan – getting Gary and Grandma to race down the aisles. I'm not concerned about the manager complaining because, based on the speed, only Matt and I can tell this is a race. Maybe a check-out girl figures out what is going on. She is laughing her head off when we reach her.

They're exhausted by the time we leave and they both struggle to get down off of the four-inch curb. A blond-haired, middle-aged woman in a wheelchair and her aide, who is pushing her, stare at Grandma and Gary without speaking. I look at their faces, something I never used to do because I was too busy getting my errands done and not wanting their sadness to interfere with my life. They seem cheerless.

I walk up to them as Gary and Grandma are discussing methods to go down the one step to the street, and ask, "Want to race?" They both look up at me like I'm some kind of crackpot. They don't say anything and I don't think they're counting to eight. I break the silence with, "Let's see who can get in the car first. You have to be fully sitting with the car door shut. We'll wait till those two get on the street level and then you're off. OK?" I sound like a referee explaining the rules for the gold medal. The woman looks up at her helper and says, "You in?" The helper nods.

I stand on the street with my mother and her cane, my son and his cane, and the woman in the wheelchair, all lined up like it is an Olympic race. Matt is holding the bag with the dishtowel. He snaps the dishtowel like it is a starter flag. He says, "Ready? Get set. Go!"

The wheelchair team speeds ahead. But their car is further away. They look like they are gloating. But they have to put the wheelchair in the vehicle for the victory. When Gary and Grandma see the wheelchair team's early lead they seem more determined than ever. Grandma takes off. (Well, it's relative. She huffs and puffs, as she carefully places the cane in front of her feet. She tries not to trip while looking up at the car and determining whether she has the wind in her 81-year-old lungs to make it.) Gary laughs so hard watching her try to walk fast that he is in last place. But I see his determination: he doesn't want to be outshined by Grandma and the strangers. He puts the cane in front of his feet and takes careful steps to make it to the car. The blonde and her helper are at their car door and Gary and Grandma are steps away from our car. Matt is cheering on Gary. The helper hustles to get the woman seated in the car. They know they have to work together to get the door closed. I hear the thud of the closed door and the helper screams out in a heavy accent, "We are winning!" Now, she has to fold up the wheelchair. While she fumbles putting the wheelchair in the trunk, Grandma arrives at our car, but isn't inside. Gary is behind but he's closing the distance.

Matt says, "Come on, Grandma! She's having trouble getting the wheelchair in the car. Just get in and close the door!"

The helper manages to shut the door then screams out "We won!" across the parking lot. I wave a thumbs-up. Grandma hears the victors' words just as she readies to close her car door, which would earn her second place. But she struggles with getting the cane inside. Instead of getting in himself, Gary opts to help Grandma close her door. As we drive off, Gary says he sees the blonde and her helper at a traffic light still laughing.

"I didn't lose, Mom," Gary says.

Is he so used to needing to perform that he feels bad about this? Does he think I am disappointed in him? I'm horrified at this thought. As my mind races through all the ways that I'm a bad mother, Gary interrupts my thoughts with, "Did you see that woman smile?"

I look in my rearview mirror and see his broad smile, the one that lights up his face and makes me melt.

"I sure did," I say.

What You Can Do Now

---

1. Make recovery fun.

There is still pain and it is a struggle to regain what you've lost, if you even can. I reset the performance bar for Gary by having him compete with Grandma and even a stranger in a wheelchair. Everyone had fun racing for the car.

2. Smile at a person in a wheelchair.

You'll both feel better.

* * *

Chapter 12
And Then a Hero Comes Along

Gary is 5'8" tall, weighs 116 pounds and looks like a rubber band stretched and ready to snap if stretched anymore. The school administration is pretty clear on Gary's return: Not so fast. The counselor fears that during classroom changes, with the crowded halls, a kid's backpack can ram into Gary's stomach by accident, opening his incision. So, the school sends tutors to our house. Sometimes three tutors a day come to catch Gary up on his class work. I have no idea what he is learning, but I watch each day pass and judge his recovery by the speed at which he is able to go downstairs and walk to the table to study. After two days, he stops walking downstairs. He glides instead. It's easier. He uses his strong arms to hold on to the banister and the wall and leaps down five stairs a time. He makes it down in three leaps.

After we've been home about two weeks, Gary announces in the middle of his biology lesson that he wants to return to school … tomorrow. He's had it with being home. When the bio tutor leaves, I tell my mom to get ready – we're going to the school. I look for any reason to keep her moving. She can rest in the car while Gary and I talk to the guidance counselor. Mrs. Peters is a seasoned, busy, high school administrator. She takes us right in. I bet she's heard it all. Her clothes are worn thin, her gray roots are an inch long next to her Lucy Ricardo red hair, and she wears no makeup. Still, she emits energy that shines brighter than the sparkly expensive necklace I am wearing from my former days as an executive. I wonder why I still bother to put it on. I don't need to impress her. She sincerely wants to help Gary. She agrees to let Gary return to school. The only stipulation is that he has to leave each class five minutes early so he can walk the halls when they are empty. He seems thrilled. As we exit her office, I notice her secretary, Ms. Lang. She sits in tight quarters in the front office of the guidance department in a wheelchair. She has MS and her work space is designed for her to be able to maneuver from the phone to the computer to the copy machine without standing up.

"I used to take walking for granted," Gary says, holding up his cane.

Mrs. Lang says, "I deal with what is handed to me."

I notice she does not say, "What doesn't kill us makes us stronger," or any other cliché. Instead she adds, "You'll be able to keep up one day and you'll always appreciate that gift."

The buzzer for the next class rings and the halls fill with students. They have so much energy. Since they are not allowed to run in the halls, their zeal is released by the volume of their voices. Gary just stares at them. He has to stay in the office until the class change ends. It gives him time to chat with Ms. Lang.

He says, "I thought I learned this lesson about appreciating the little things when I was in South Africa."

"You were in South Africa?"

"Yeah, I won a contest with National Geographic kids. They were looking for explorers. I was one of 15 kids out of 5,000 to go."

"Wow, that's amazing." Ms. Lang says.

The phone rings and she picks it up. She sends a quick e-mail about the call. When she's done, she looks up at Gary, who is ready to burst wanting to finish the story.

"Yeah, I dove with a great white shark and I saw lions mating but nothing left an impression on me like the kids there. They took us to a township."

Mrs. Lang seems interested so he continues.

"They live in houses the size of garden sheds. They have no

electricity. They have no running water. Ten people can live in one shed. But you know what?"

"What?"

"They seemed so joyful. I got to play soccer with them. They didn't have a field or sneakers. It seemed like the whole town came for the game and sang songs and cheered. They beat us. We had sneakers, but they had spirit."

I interrupt Gary's telling of the story. "National Geographic let each child take one parent on the trip. In the township, I was over-whelmed with sadness from how little they had; mothers with no shoes carrying babies. Forget about washing machines. They walk four miles a day for water. The township went on for acres and acres. I never felt so helpless and overwhelmed with so much suffering."

The phone rings again. Now I cannot wait to tell her the rest of the story. I stand by the desk as she patiently explains to some-body that it is too late for a student to drop a course. She takes a message for Mrs. Peters to get back to the parent. She looks up at me so I continue.

"Gary said we had to help them. I didn't know what to say to him. How in the world could we help these people? I felt hopeless. Just as I was about to tell Gary there was no way to make an impact on so much poverty, you won't believe what happened. I feel funny saying it, but it's true."

I don't want her to think I'm some crackpot but, I sense by her expression, she sincerely wants to know and won't judge me. "Tell me," Mrs. Lang says.

"I looked up into the blue sky. I couldn't believe what I saw. I did a double take. It was still there: a rainbow. The publisher of the magazine, standing next to me, saw the rainbow too. It wasn't rain-ing, but there it was. I couldn't believe it. I felt hope. I'd never felt such a transition before. I told Gary we'd find a way."

Gary exclaims, "We sure did. When I got back to school in the fall, my principal, Mr. Harris, got a call from this man, Mark

Grashow, who wanted to help kids in Africa. Mr. Harris put me on the phone with Mr. Grashow. The next day he came to my school! I showed him my pictures of the kids in Africa and said I wanted to help them. He wanted to do the same thing! He needed supplies for two libraries he was building in Zimbabwe. He asked the principal if we could do a drive to collect stuff."

Gary tells Mrs. Lang about how the principal seemed a little unsure of the guy, and how the guy then pulled out a book – "Giving" by Bill Clinton. It was the same book I'd given to Gary when we got back from our trip.

Gary says, "He opened the book and this guy Mark is in chapter four in Bill Clinton's book. It's about how he gives to the people of Africa. My principal approved the drive on the spot. In two weeks we collected enough stuff for two schools. We sent almost a shipping container full of stuff, even clothes and shoes and sports equipment. Now I'm trying to get water."

One water pump can supply 2,600 people and costs $14,000, he tells her. He doesn't have a clue about how he's going to get the money.

With the halls now empty we leave. My boots echo on the hard tile as I walk at a snail's pace with Gary back to the car. Gary seems embarrassed by the racket of my boots. I am embarrassed, too, but for a different reason. I take off my necklace and stuff it in my handbag.

Gary says he's starving so we wake Grandma from her catnap in the car and go out to lunch. Gary wolfs down the food, Japanese again, but at a new restaurant. I am thrilled to see him eating. He is skin and bones. We finish eating just after 1 p.m. and Gary looks tired. I drive him and Grandma home to rest. With both of them sleeping, I relish a couple of hours of being able to work. I go to my basement office, open my e-mails and see 57 that I still need to respond to, a manageable number. Gary returning to school will mean our lives are getting back on track. I count the days to tennis tryouts and figure that if Gary starts training in three weeks he should be able to try out for the team. Also, the tutors have him almost caught up. I pound through and respond to about 25 e-mails. I'm flying without an elephant in sight. I take a break and microwave a cup of hot chocolate, with extra marshmallows, and stir. Some marshmallows stick on the spoon and I love the melted sweet gooeyness. The house is quiet and I let the heat of the hot chocolate warm me up. I go back downstairs to finish up the rest of the e-mails. Before I know it, it's 5 p.m. I venture upstairs to check on Gary. I see him sitting up in bed. The painful expression on his face shocks me.

"Mom, my stomach hurts," he says.

"Is it the same as before?"

"No," he says. "I think I have a stomachache."

Let's see, he ate a bowl of rice, two California rolls, and a bento box with chicken teriyaki, green beans and dumplings. No wonder his stomach aches!

"Well, you did eat a lot. And I've heard there is a stomach bug going around. I think you'll stay home one more day tomorrow."

"OK," he says without putting up much protest, which immediately worries me.

I call the pediatrician's office and they confirm there is a stomach bug going around and that lots of kids are throwing up, which is what Gary is doing now. They suggest he should rest.

Gary is up all night. The next day he tries to rest. At night again, he confides that the pain is getting worse and worse, worse than the peeing pain! The constant cramps won't subside and he can't sleep. He just crouches and holds his side. I rub his back as he throws up for the umpteenth time. Around midnight I see this green brownish stuff come out. I've never seen anything that color and texture from my insides. I call the pediatrician's office and I am told to bring him to the Norwalk emergency room.

I tiptoe into my mother's room to tell her. Gary is in the worst pain I've ever seen. He says it feels like there are spasms in his intestines that won't stop. He is beyond crying. He just tries to breathe through each cramp. He sits in the car and does not speak. Instead, it is as if he's entered a soundproof room and I am banished from him. I drive to the E.R., terrified. I know Gary usually finds comfort in my strength but it's gone. My hands shake on the steering wheel.

Gary staggers into the E.R. holding his side. I give my insurance card to the check-in desk and hear a booming voice giving orders. I look up to see who is so confident. The E.R. doctor on call is a relatively young man with dark wavy hair. He is a little too good-looking and wears his white shirt a little too snug, underscoring that he spends time at the gym. It seems like he hasn't experienced the weight of the world yet, he just lifts them. I don't like him.

I hear him ordering around the nurses and see him flirting with an especially pretty blonde in a skirt. No one looks familiar from our last visit – only three weeks ago – and no one seems to care. My skepticism, I am sure, is seen on my face.

Gary is placed in the same partitioned area as the last time. This time, the pain doesn't subside. Gary whispers that even if he wanted to do homework, like last time, he couldn't. These are the first words I hear him say since leaving the house. I'm sick to my stomach.

I try to comfort him with, "It's OK." But he's not hearing anything. It's like he is having labor pains but much, much worse. The nurses take his vitals and within minutes Doctor Youngbuck, as I nickname him, stops by. He suggests a pain medication that he tells me is powerful. I can't even pronounce its name.

Gary yells, "Give it to me! I can't take this anymore."

I don't ask about the risks of the medication or its spelling so I can Google it. In my helpless state, I just have to trust this doctor whom I don't know and have never seen before, and hope that he'll care for my son. The doctor takes a syringe and injects Gary's arm. Gary feels better instantly, almost too fast. I don't even think the doctor is done with the injection before I see Gary's face muscles relax. It seems almost the same way I felt after being in labor for hours and finally getting the epidural. Once the injection empties,

Gary sighs with relief. As he lies on the bed, he smiles at me. The doctor announces he needs to take a CT scan to see what is causing the pain. With Gary having a little respite, I find the strength to think again and find it fascinating that no one tracks how much radiation this child is getting. My instincts say that it's too much. I challenge the doctor about the CT scan and ask if there's any other way to see what is happening.

"Yes, CT scans do have a lot of radiation. A CT scan can be similar to 1,000 X-rays." He pauses. "We don't need the full definition at this point. We can do an X-ray instead."

Instantly, my opinion of him starts to change. I like that he is flexible. I smile. I don't know if he noticed but I start to trust him a little. I wonder to myself, if I did not speak up would they just have automatically done a CT scan? No one has asked me how many other CT scans Gary's had. The X-ray reveals a blockage but the doctor can't tell what is causing it. He instructs the staff to insert an NG tube into Gary's stomach so he won't have to keep throwing up. The tube will automatically empty Gary's stomach. The tube is a big, thick plastic cylinder. It needs to go up Gary's nose and down his esophagus into his stomach. Gary is awake for this entire procedure. The nurse sits Gary up and starts to shove it in. It's too big to fit and Gary is miserable. She tries again. They have to slide the tube past his gagging response and keep funneling it down into his stomach. The tube causes him to reflex and dry heave. Gary clutches onto the rails of the gurney as they keep pushing more and more tube into his body until it reaches his stomach. The instant the procedure is done Gary demands that they take it out. It doesn't matter how many times the nurse explains that he can't have anything else go in his stomach. I've never seen him complain relentlessly.

The doctors say that Gary needs to be transferred to Children's Hospital in Hartford – immediately – since it is so soon after his last surgery. As he waits to be released from the E.R., the pain medicine wears off. Gary looks exhausted from his sleepless night. He begs them to remove the tube but they refuse. Gary blurts out, "Then give me another hit."

I'm terrified. His choice of words seem like an addict's. Is this like seeing my kid on heroin? There is no talking to him. He is demanding the drug. Watching Gary plead for another hit makes me realize how fast I can lose my child. With Gary's commotion, the doctor comes in and says that the painkiller was very potent. He will not give him more.

"Then take out the NG tube. I hate it!"

"No," the doctor states. "You need it for the transfer to Hartford Hospital."

In the end, they give him something. I don't know what they give him to calm him down, but it is something. Gary settles down but I can tell the pain didn't go away. I'm in a daze. It is the middle of the night. They are arranging for an ambulance to transfer us.

"You'll have to move your car from the hospital emergency entrance before the ambulance will transport you and your son to Hartford hospital," a nurse says.

I look at Gary hooked up to the I.V., and with a tube coming out of his nose. He is holding the tube almost as if he wants to pull it out and just go home. There is nothing for me to say except the obvious.

"Honey, I have to move the car. I'll be right back."

"Yeah."

I dash through the double glass doors as rain pounds on the pavement. It's a relentless rain. The ambulance is scheduled to leave in 15 minutes.

"You have an umbrella?" I ask the burly security guard.

"Nope."

"How about a garbage bag?"

"Nope," he says.

Instead of bolting to the car to stay dry, I walk. I feel the rain soak my hair and pour over my face. I hear the clap of thunder and it sounds furious. I look up at the sky, feel my mascara run down my face, and shake my head, like a dog drying herself off. I open the car door, not caring about getting the seats wet, and I turn on the ignition. I move the car to the long-term parking lot. The windshield wipers race back and forth. I can barely see the parking space lines. I pick a spot at the furthest end. I don't know when I'll be back to pick up the car. It's pouring even heavier as I get out of the car. A lightning bolt slams down and at the same moment, I hear a huge roar of thunder, right above me. It's the kind of closeness that usually makes me run for cover. But, I'm not scared of being hit. There is no way I am going to be hit. I just know life can't be that cruel. I need strength, not fear, to care for my child. The rain pours on my face as I make my way back to the emergency room. My sweatshirt and socks soak up so much water that I feel like I am carrying the weight of two of me. I glance at my watch. It's 3 a.m. With no one around, I scream purposely and slowly at the top of my lungs, to the point that my throat feels raw.

"I have nothing left!"

I want God to know. Right after I finish the sentence another bolt of lightning and thunder occur, as if in response. I stand in the middle of the parking lot and I don't even flinch. I scream even louder and slower.

"I. HAVE. NOTHING. LEFT."

I walk to the waiting ambulance.

Gary is on a stretcher in the back with an EMT by his side. As usual, I sit next to the driver, a not-even-25-year-old with more tattoos than birthdays. He is blasting heavy metal music that seems to keep rhythm with the pounding of the rain against the windshield. I hate the music and normally would speak up about it but I don't care anymore. This is my reality. This is my son's reality. The driver pulls onto I-95 and is driving too fast, especially in the rainstorm. For the last couple of miles an 18-wheeler pulls up alongside the ambulance. I look at the truck driver and he seems to be from the same mold as my driver. I think they are racing! The paramedic, in the back, yells over the music that the medications are working; Gary's vitals are normal.

The pounding music, the pelting of the raindrops against the windshield and the few inches between my passenger seat and the huge truck as we race along the highway makes me even more terrified. I silently tell God that if this is the end, it's OK. It's in Your hands now, I tell him, and close my eyes and wait for the crash.

The driver interrupts my prayers with his first words to me since we pulled onto the highway. I am in my own world and it takes me a while to hear him. He repeats the question louder and I look up at him.

"You like this music?"

"Not really," I say, grateful. "I'm tired. Something quieter please."

He changes the radio station. I can't believe my ears. I hear Mariah Carey belt out "Hero."

> *"And then a hero comes along,*
> *with the strength to carry on*
> *and you cast your fears aside*
> *and you know you can survive.*
> *So when you feel like hope is gone,*
> *look inside you and be strong*
> *and you will finally see the truth*
> *that a hero lies in you."*

Mariah eases me back to reality. Out the window, the 18-wheeler is barreling toward the exit. We are not going to crash. It's not the end. The driver keeps talking and tells me that originally he took the job for his beer money, but he's discovered he likes helping people. I see beyond the snake tattoo on his neck and notice his warm smile. I smile back.

Mariah continues,

"Lord knows dreams are to follow
but don't let anyone tear them away.
Hold on, there will be tomorrow
in time you'll find the way."

I wonder if Gary is listening. This is his song. It was the number one song the day he was born and I play it for him all the time! I turn around to look. Gary's eyes are open. He is quiet and seems as comfortable as can be expected. Maybe he already believes what she is singing. When I turn back to look at the front windshield, I notice it's stopped raining. We travel the next hour without needing windshield wipers. I look up and say thank you. I even nod off for a bit.

What You Can Do Now

---

1. Take a moment for yourself.

I enjoyed a cup of hot chocolate with extra marshmallows and allowed the heat of the cup to warm me up.

2. Don't assume the doctors communicate with each other.

When Gary started throwing up, it didn't occur to me that it could be because of the surgery three weeks earlier. I did not bring up the surgery when talking with the nurse. I assumed the pediatrician would have connected the symptom instead of saying it was the stomach flu. I learned it is my job to over communicate and repeat the obvious information about the patient.

3. Be honest with yourself.

It's OK to feel overwhelmed. Acknowledge it. Feel it. Say it. I found when I was at my rawest, I saw and heard things differently. Be open to your new perspective.

* * *

Chapter 13
Ask Why, Say No

The driver nudges me awake and I hear the back double-doors open. I know the drill well: The paramedic and the driver take Gary out of the ambulance and transfer him to the intake nurse. I used to think the ambulance crew seemed too preoccupied with paperwork during the transfer, but now I get it. It's the official handoff. It's the protocol. I stumble out of the ambulance, which is high off the ground. I look for my handbag holding the entrance ticket, my insurance card, but I can't find it. I know Gary is in responsible hands but without my handbag – and the card – I'll be unable to answer the first question they ask. Panic creeps in. Did I leave it in the Norwalk E.R.? It's dark in the ambulance. I search between the driver's seat and mine. I look by my feet. I feel for my bag under the passenger seat and I find it, tucked away under there.

I stumble over to the triage desk, where Gary's information is already in the system. As expected, one of her first questions is about my insurance: "Has it changed?" In three weeks? I know it's protocol to ask the question, but how about a little compassion, like saying, "Oh, I'm so sorry you are back here so soon," and then returning to protocol? As much as I love routine, I hate that I've learned the steps to *this* process.

Because Gary arrived by ambulance there's no waiting to be seen. Gary is holding the NG tubing with one hand and looks ready to yank it out. He keeps repeating "Get it out!" sounding like a heavy metal artist screeching a song without any lyric development, just a heavy beat. Gary does not miss a beat. "Get it out!" "Get it out!"

"Get it out!"

A seasoned nurse replies, "They won't take it out. It has to stay in until we're directed otherwise."

Gary screams his song directly at her. I don't think she likes heavy metal either. She quickly departs, leaving me as the sole audience. After an eternity of Gary on automatic repeat the nurse returns and Gary quiets down to hear her news.

"The doctor wants to take an X-ray of the tube to make sure it is positioned correctly in his stomach. They need to confirm Norwalk's E.R. procedure."

She has got to be kidding me. Where else could the tube be? Is there another path from his esophagus that I don't know about? We need an X-ray to find this out? When my husband had pre-cancerous nodules on his thyroid as an adult, a doctor-friend speculated that Steve had probably had too many X-rays as a child. My father-in-law says that my hypochondriac mother-in-law took Steve routinely for X-rays to check his lungs for bronchitis. Now, Steve has had thyroid surgery and parathyroid surgery. That pediatrician might be long gone, but my husband lives with the results of too much testing. There is no way my kid is going to be so over-radiated that he ends up with cancer in 30 years. My exhaustion and skepticism lead me to shout "No!"

I never shout and Gary looks up at me. The nurse restates, as if I didn't hear her the first time, "We need to know that the NG tube is positioned correctly." Maybe she thinks if she just keeps repeating the same thing my response will change. I tell her, "Look, I am finding it very difficult to believe that the only way you can tell if this is in correctly is with an X-ray." I am firm, not even trying to be friendly. I look like a dried out drowned rat and feel the same. My wet sneakers squeak as I walk closer to her.

"That's what the doctor wants," she says.

I get it. The protocol train provides her comfort with a clear track to follow. There need to be consistent processes. There need to be rules of authority. There shouldn't be mavericks running loose. But this does prevent people from thinking for themselves.

"Look, there will be no X-ray," I say. "Find another way."

"So, may I state this correctly? You are refusing medical treatment for your son."

Here we go again. Only this time, I see the clearness of her question and guilt-producing tactic. Either I change my mind or, if I do not, the hospital will document my response and protect itself legally. I don't even find it hard to muster up the courage to say, "No X-ray. Find another way."

She leaves the room. Gary screams that he doesn't care about another X-ray. He just wants this NG tube out. To him, the point I am making about excessive radiation seems to be missing his point. Gary switches to the silent treatment. I don't know which I hate more, this or his heavy metal version of "I hate it." Time could not be moving any slower. The nurse finally opens the door. She repeats that the doctors wanted an X-ray to be done in the E.R., but since I am refusing treatment, they will be moving Gary, now, to a room upstairs.

She looks at Gary and says, "The E.R. doctor said the tube stays in." She is letting us both know I lost the battle. But, I'm glad Gary didn't get another dose of radiation. The floor nurse points us to our new home, for I have no idea how long, and I notice that the day bed seems to at least have a better mattress: one single cushion, no sagging possible. Why would the hospital even have day beds with separate cushions, when there is a better way? I bet no one in purchasing has ever slept on one of those other beds.

Gary's new nurse looks like she graduated yesterday. I hold back my question wondering if Gary is her first patient. I know how important nurses are and I don't want to piss her off right away. Maybe later, but I should at least try to be nice.

"I understand they are concerned about whether the NG tube is placed properly," she says, smiling.

"Yeah," I say. Now I'm answering with the monosyllables.

"I understand you said no getting an X-ray?"

"Yeah."

"I have an idea. I learned in nursing school that the pH of the stomach is in the one-to-three range. I bet I can get some pH papers and then I can test some of the stuff coming out of the tube."

I can't believe there can be a solution as simple as this. "Really?" I say.

"Sure! Let me get the papers." She races out of the room.

Gary, who hasn't spoken to me since we arrived in the E.R., reiterates that his issue is not the X-ray or the placement of the tube. He wants the tube out. If the X-ray reveals that the tube is in the wrong place and they remove the tube then getting the X-ray is well worth the test. To him, I am missing the entire point and therefore I am a bad mother. I'm acting like a radiation maniac. In less than two minutes, the nurse is back and she goes to the bag that collects the stuff from Gary's stomach and puts some cloudy gel-like liquid in a cup. Without speaking, she takes a pH strip and places it in the cup.

Gary looks over and she brings the color guide over to him. She says if it turns in the reddish area we know that the pH level is in range and that means the stuff is from his stomach and the tube is in properly. It takes seconds for the strip to turn scarlet. So, the weird liquid is the acid from his stomach. I am thrilled but also perplexed. How come they couldn't do this in the E.R.? Isn't this cheaper than an X-ray? I know it is safer. And faster.

As I stand by Gary's side looking at the pH strip, the door opens. A middle-aged man wearing a white medical jacket, but otherwise unremarkable, introduces himself as Dr. Hughes. I've never met him before, but I know his reputation in the IBD world: stellar. He wasn't taking any new patients when his partner, Dr. Simmon, agreed to work with Gary. He is one of the reasons we picked Dr. Simmon. Dr. Hughes is the doctor that Dr. Stark called when she put Gary on steroids the last time Gary was hospitalized. My antenna goes up.

Gary starts to screech his "No tube" song. Dr. Hughes looks at me and Gary and says he understands. He tells us he'll go to discuss its removal with another doctor. As he walks out the door, he reassures us that he'll be back soon.

About two hours later, Dr. Hughes returns, a nurse by his side. He smiles at Gary and tells the nurse to remove the NG tube. The nurse walks over to Gary, who, for the first time since the middle of last night, smiles. He sits up as she yanks the tube and pulls and pulls and pulls. In seconds the NG tube is out. Gary thanks Dr. Hughes, who leaves the room with the nurse.

That's it?

Gary loves this victory and so do I, but for different reasons: He got the NG tube removed and I avoided him enduring another X-ray. I high-five Gary, but wonder why the change in course. The cramps are still there. What is going on? What's the plan? I don't feel like I know anything. Steve is driving up to the hospital from New Jersey. He's stopping by the house to bring us our toothbrushes and his T-shirt for me to sleep in. The whirlwind starts up again. My cellphone rings continuously. Our friends and relatives are shocked that Gary is back here. They automatically say they are sending a card. I am hoping to be home before the cards arrive, but who knows?

A doctor, who gives me his name and who I might have seen before but I am too exhausted to remember, enters the room and goes over to Gary and quickly looks him over. The doctor turns to me and says, "We have to do a U.G.I., a small bowel study."

I must look perplexed because he continues, "We want to see if they can see the blockage."

I look at him and explain that Gary is the patient, talk to him. I'm not sure why I seem to have to explain this to each of the doctors; they are not doing this U.G.I. thing on me. He needs to get Gary's buy-in. He walks over to Gary and keeps the conversation simple. As he talks, my mind is racing. Why didn't anyone suspect a blockage when Gary was throwing up for two days? He'd just had surgery! Now, I feel guilty. Could the blockage have been avoided if I'd reacted more quickly? What was that disgusting green stuff? I am barely listening to the doctor when I hear him mention, "You'll need to drink barium." The "B" word. Just hearing the word brings back the memory of three years ago. Gary takes a deep breath. He holds his stomach that is still cramping. He looks up at the doctor and says, "If I drink the barium, you'll be able to see if there is a blockage and then get it out so the pain goes away?"

"Yes," the doctor responds. Doctors only answer the questions you ask.

"Let's get started," Gary exclaims, with the same enthusiasm of someone shouting out, "Play ball!"

He must be in so much pain if even barium doesn't seem that bad. "The attendant will take you downstairs," the doctor says. "You'll have to drink it and wait four hours for it to go through your system. We will take a look as it travels in your intestines. You'll stay by the X-ray machine so we can take pictures at different intervals to see where the blockage is."

Ugh. X-rays. Again. But there's no way around these. I keep my mouth shut.

"Great," Gary responds. He actually sounds sincere.

Gary is maturing before my eyes. He doesn't bitch and complain about the stuff. I don't have to give him the lecture about letting them help. Or the other lecture that reminds him that next week this will be over, tomorrow it will be over, this evening it will be over. It's four hours. No, this time, Gary already has the skills. He stands up, unplugs his monitor from behind the bed and grabs the I.V. cords and says, "Which way to the X-ray room?"

I follow Gary in his hospital gown and the attendant to the elevator. We pass the visitors in street clothes in the hall. We pass the fish tank with the Nemo fish, the one where Grandma broke down and cried. This place holds our family memories. I see a new crop of moms with their toddlers using the fish as a distraction. If they have Crohn's, I know the path they are on. But in this moment, the kids seem happy looking for Nemo.

Gary goes to the reception desk to let them know he is here and the nurse tells us to wait. We spend four hours on couches against the wall in the glaring corridor. The linoleum floors echo the steps of families whose loved ones need X-rays. I try to rest my head on the wooden arm of the couch. My head hurts. I try to put my feet up but the couches are too small for me to lie down on. These couches are too uncomfortable for me even in my physical and emotional exhausted state to relax. Forget Steve. They are not designed for the over six-foot set. Who picked these things? Did they ever pull an all-nighter on them alongside a kid in pain?

Gary takes the "chocolate syrup" from the nurse. He is told he has less than one hour to drink it. He is tired too and in too much pain to complain. In between sips Gary tries to relax. The cramps have not subsided and he is exhausted. At least he's not throwing up.

Steve finds us in the hall. He must have rushed; he looks like a panting dog. He hugs Gary and gently, quickly, kisses me. I point to the couch for him to sit down and Gary takes another sip of barium. He doesn't say anything and Steve just gives him the thumbs up sign. Then, Steve moves the wires from the I.V. machines so they won't get tangled as Gary tries to lie down on the couch. Gary puts his head on the wooden arm rest. He tries to put his feet up on the couch. He turns his head. He moves his feet. Gary is in his hospital gown with rubber soled socks. People try to ignore him as they pass by on their way to the X-ray room.

Steve is tired and tries to get comfortable. No way will he find a comfortable position here, though. He is a half foot taller than Gary. This is almost funny to watch. The wooden arm barely supports Steve's neck and his head droops off. He looks like an upside down V. All three of us must look miserable. Occasionally, a pretty nurse comes over to see how Gary is doing drinking the barium. He says, "At least I don't have to pee," and then takes a big swig.

Finally, after hours, a man comes out from one of the rooms and says there is a place where Gary can stay while he is doing the barium study. The man and a nurse move Gary to a stretcher and wheel him to a room. They even have chairs for Steve and me, the kind with a high back so our necks don't snap when we nod off. They even turn the lighting down. We don't have to be in the middle of a hall. As Gary finally closes his eyes waiting for the next X-ray, I wonder who designs these processes? If it takes four hours for the barium study, why in the world does it make sense for an in-house patient to have to wait in the hall? Hasn't anyone in this place ever needed these services? It's like someone designed a train to get to a place, but never rode it.

At least Gary can rest and wait as the barium travels through his system. Occasionally they wake him and take a snapshot. At one point they come in and tell us, "We see the blockage. We need to operate because something is blocking the food from passing." Something is stuck in his intestines, but the only thing that went in there is food. In my heart, I know it is all that rice he ate at the Japanese restaurant. I bet the cramps kept squeezing the rice until it was like a brick and now it is stuck. No one tells me otherwise and I don't hear any other medical facts. Gary is thrilled they see something. It's further proof that he is not imagining this. Gary's spasms have not stopped. It's like day three of labor. It's Saturday, I think. I've lost track of time. Many doctors come in and press on his stomach. I keep thinking about all that rice Gary ate. He got sick a couple of hours after that meal. The doctors don't ask me or Gary about what he has eaten. This is a real sore point with me. He is a Crohn's patient. Crohn's is a digestive disorder. But talking to the doctors about food is like talking to a brick wall. Now is not the time for a debate. I already know the answer. Without more data, I stick to my simple, non-medical, just logical explanation, "Yes, the blockage is the rice from Gary's lunch before he got sick."

To prove my point, I ask them how long it would take for the lunch to digest.

"Four hours," a doctor responds.

Bingo. He started cramping exactly four hours after he ate. This confirms it to me. There is a bunch of rice stuck. But, they keep saying he needs surgery to remove the blockage. Gary is lying on the bed and the cramps are relentless. He is in massive pain, much worse than the peeing pain from last time. He just wants the spasms to stop. I want that, too, but one thing I am learning is I have a voice. I've already seen that when I speak up, I can help Gary. As hard as this is for me, I need to make sure we choose the right course of action.

"Doctor, if he has surgery won't he go through the same recovery process again?"

"Yes."

"He'll miss more school; he won't be able to walk, which he just started to do."

"Yes."

"He won't train for tennis?"

"That's correct. But if this were my child, I would be doing the surgery right now," Dr. Hughes practically yells at me.

Coming off my X-ray victory just a couple of hours earlier, I am not relenting easily. I think this place has helped me develop immunity to the guilt tactic, the unwritten protocol method to get the train moving in the doctor's direction.

"What else can you do if I am right and it's the rice that is stuck?" I ask.

"Well, we can go up his anus and flush it out. It is uncomfortable for the patient and I would not recommend it. Plus it can be humiliating for boys," Dr. Hughes says to me.

"Let me understand." I pause for a breath and think to myself that they have an alternative. If I didn't ask they were not going to tell me. I continue, "You can try to flush it out like a roto-rooter?"

Dr. Hughes smiles at my analogy but uses medical terms to

describe the process which seems to me to say it is like unplugging a drain pipe with liquid.

"So if this works, he would not need surgery? He would feel better, no new incisions and the recovery time is much less?"

"Yes. But he needs surgery."

I walk over to the couch to give myself a moment to think. The doctor's response seems strange. Normally, they add in a gray area by saying some percentage of chance or they explain it with so many medical terms I feel lost. Not this time. The only answer is surgery. How do they know it is not the rice creating the blockage? So far, I've learned that I can lead a medical team to look for options. They listen. Each time it's worked. Like Gary didn't need steroids before the last surgery, he didn't need a CT scan to see the blockage in the E.R. and he didn't need an X-ray to locate the NG tube placement. I pushed and we found a less insidious method to treat the problem. Why should I stop now?

"Find out if you can try this, please," I ask.

They walk out of the room, stating they have to make a few calls.

I wish Gary's loud moans were for added effect, but he is in real pain and just wants it fixed. I walk over to him. He pulls my sweater so that my face is an inch from his. He is furious. I am the only one he can take his anger out on.

"You should just listen to them," he boils. "I can't take these spasms anymore."

"Gary, do you understand that if they can just do this roto-root-er thing, you will be back at school? You can play tennis? Don't you think it's worth a shot before they go and open up your belly again?" I plead.

He releases my sweater.

I continue, "Hopefully, they will come back and say they will try the roto-rooter approach."

"Mom, I don't want to have anal sex," Gary says.

Ahh, the real objection. "It's not sex, Gary. It's a medical procedure and I understand it seems invasive to you. We can ask if it hurts, OK?"

"OK." Gary tries to rest and closes his eyes. It's like he is so used to the pain, he can rest through it, or maybe the exhaustion overcomes everything.

I spend the time waiting for the doctor's return ranting about nutrition and Crohn's to whichever nurse comes into Gary's room. It's a digestive disease. How come they don't ask anything about what he eats? It doesn't pass my common sense test. The nurses listen to me. They don't agree with me nor do they disagree. I worked for a big company, too. I get it. But, I sense they support me pushing the doctors to challenge protocol.

It feels like an hour later when two doctors return to the room, Dr. Hughes and a new doctor. Dr. Hughes lets me know they have arranged for a doctor to do the roto-rooter procedure and the room is being made ready.

"Thank you." I beam. They say they hope it works. They walk over to Gary and one of them says, "Good luck. We will be standing by in the hospital awaiting the results." They quickly leave.

Moments later, the attendant comes to move Gary's bed downstairs. The door frame is at a 90-degree angle to the bed. The nurse appears from behind the bed, where she bends down and pushes the bed away to unplug Gary's pump. Now, she needs help to get the bed into position to squeeze through the door. I watch them maneuver the bed with Gary, the I.V. tubes and the pumping machine and I wish the door frame were even one more inch wider. As an engineer, this kills me. It would be so much easier for the attendant to position the bed in the room without having to get the bed near perfectly aligned to pass through the door. After weeks in this hospital I notice these things. I wait until the bed finally makes it through the door frame and comment, "I bet you both wish they changed this set-up."

"What?"

"The electrical outlets, they are behind the bed. Wouldn't it be easier for you if they were on the side wall?" I say.

They both laugh. "You've been here a while."

I see the challenges in their work from a user perspective, not some hierarchical boss just telling them what to do and not asking their input or understanding the basic struggles of the job. They have every right to be frustrated. How many times a day do they have to overcome skinny door frames? It shouldn't be a challenge to get the bed out of the room. With all that energy spent on bed manipulation, it's hard to focus on the patient. I bet that is one reason why Gary and other patients become a widget in their machine.

On the first floor, Gary lies in bed and is greeted by another new doctor who looks like many of the rest of them: same middle-aged crow's feet, same thinning hair, and same slight build. I wonder if all the moms seem the same to him: exhausted, nervous and tense. The same way I don't even try to learn his name is the same way he doesn't even ask me mine.

The room seems well lit but feels dark. There are no windows in here, just a big monitor and stainless steel equipment. Once again the room is filled with strangers. It's not clear who does what. I don't think anyone introduces themselves to me. They are busy setting up equipment. Two people go over to Gary and tell him they need to move him onto a small bed. Gary even volunteers to help move himself from one bed to another instead of being lifted on sheets and slid over. Gary hoists himself by his arms and slides his rump over. I watch as he works through the pain.

A new nurse introduces herself to Gary. Gary asks only one question: "Does it hurt?"

"Not really," she says. "We are going to insert a tube up your rectum and then flush a liquid up. Then at the end of the procedure you will expel the liquid. You will feel some pressure."

Gary rolls in any direction he is told. He doesn't complain. He does not say anything. I watch the procedure from a corner of the room. It's quiet as the doctor pumps liquid in. It feels like about 15 minutes and the doctor announces it's over. He tells Gary to poop.

Gary lies on the bed with a nurse holding a bucket by him. I hear the fluid rushing from his body. I pray that the rice comes with it. Gary squeezes his face. He tries and tries to push it out. I squeeze the arm chair with each push. The rice does not dislodge. I'm heartbroken. I look up at Gary. Neither one of us says it, but I think we both have the same thought: at least we tried. He doesn't look angry. He looks resolved for surgery. I appreciate the doctor's support. Within minutes one doctor tells me, "We are going to do emergency surgery."

Everything takes forever in the hospital, yet they are already for surgery *now*? Somehow I feel like they knew what the outcome would be all along. That's preposterous though, isn't it? They wouldn't go through this whole procedure knowing it was a façade. Would they? A doctor in the roto-rooter room mentions something about the blockage being caused by "adhesions." I don't know what he means and I don't think I've ever heard this term before. No one ever mentioned anything about adhesions.

Gary says something like, "I told you I needed surgery. The doctors know what they are doing, Mom. You've got to trust them."

What You Can Do Now

---

1. *The two most important steps you can take as an advocate:*
a. Ask WHY
b. Say NO

Only when you are convinced that you are following the best course of action should you say YES and feel good about your decision.

2. *Understand that no option may seem ideal.*

Many times you have to choose between bad and worse. Know that you did your best.

3. *Respect the doctors.*

I found it easier to agree to disagree. I accepted that they had the medical knowledge and the final word because I needed them to help my son.

* * *

Chapter 14

Discovering the Root Cause

The attendant maneuvers Gary on his gurney back into the elevator and to his sixth-floor room. Surgery again. I don't understand this. Gary hasn't fully recovered from his first surgery and neither have I. The room is a whirlwind again with nurses trying to comfort us and promising that once surgery is over Gary will feel great. How can they say this? He's barely walking from the first surgery. I stop listening. As the doctors come in to brief us, I just stare. I don't think I ask any questions. Steve signs the release forms.

An attendant arrives and leads the way to the third floor admitting area of the O.R. Steve walks on one side of the bed and I on the other, each of us holding Gary's hands. Only in the elevator do we separate. I don't say anything. I don't notice anything. I am beaten. I feel like a cog in a machine that will just spit me out when it's done with me.

In the dark admitting area Gary lies in bed waiting for the anesthesiologist to brief him. I feel so weak I can't even stand up. A nurse brings me a chair. She knows. I sit down and cannot hold back my tears. Gary watches me cry. Steve stands next to me, silent. He looks exhausted and defeated. His skin looks as gray as his hair. We wait for the doctor.

I am suddenly surrounded by new people telling me who they are, what their job is and that Gary will be all right. One person says she remembers Gary from the other week. The only thing I hear is Gary telling the anesthesiologist that he just wants the pain to stop and he'll do anything they want at this point.

They roll him away to surgery and a piece of my heart rolls with him. The first operation I understood. They had to remove intestine and a fistula on his bladder. The fistula caused a hole in his bladder and they repaired it. This time, I don't know what they're trying to accomplish. I don't know what "adhesions" are. I don't know why he's in such pain. We have to wait hours to find out if they can fix him, again.

We take the elevator to the second floor, the hospital cafeteria, the rocket to nowhere. The cafeteria is almost empty. It's around 7 p.m. on Saturday. I know that the doctors try to get most patients released by Friday. I never knew illness takes weekends off.

Just the die-hards, the people with really sick kids, are here. What a horrible place to eat dinner on a Saturday night. I don't see a soul smiling. Not even the wall murals of space travel let my mind wander to a happier place. Stuck here, I focus on Steve. He looks like this ordeal is about to break his back. He needs to eat. He needs some attention. We bring our trays filled with salad for me and a burger for him back to a table directly under the skylight. A yellow triangular sign on our table reminds diners about some upcoming event. I take another yellow tri-fold from an adjoining table and place it in our table's center. "Steve, it's our pretend candle lights," I say trying to brighten the mood. He smiles and takes my hand but he is crying. We sit under the stars with our pretend candles. In between the silence, Steve eats a bit of the burger or a French fry. Other than to squeeze his hand I don't know how to help my big, strong husband. Finally, Steve breaks the silence.

"We'll do whatever it takes to help Gary," he says.

"We will," I say.

I couldn't love him any more at this instant. We are married 21 years. It's a cliché that love grows stronger, but right now I know this is true. I love that Steve doesn't lament about Gary's future. Or that he's pissed off to be back in this hospital. He is not ranting and raving about doctor incompetence or how unfair this is. He is not showing his bravado by finding fault with others to show how great he is. When I said, "Yes, I'll marry you" at the age of 24, after dating Steve for only four months, I didn't know that the glimpse of Steve's character that I fell in love with would be so critical to surviving life's ups and downs. I didn't even think about life's ups and downs. For better, for worse – how bad could it be? To me, Steve was a great guy, fun, hard-working, funny and not a complainer. He was and still is good looking. But, now, I know, there is a "for worse" and how we handle our life's obstacles is how we make things, "for better."

I love that Steve has taught me through the years to live in the moment. He has never told me this, never put it in words, but I watched him appreciate the moment so many times that it has rubbed off on me. When I read "The Tao of Pooh," by Benjamin Hoff, I discovered the extent of Steve's wisdom. Hoff explains the eastern philosophy of Taoism using Winnie the Pooh characters. He puts Winnie the Pooh as the highest level of being because Pooh just lives in the moment. When Pooh is hungry he eats. If no food is available he finds some. He is simple-minded. Pooh is a great example of *wei wu wei*, the Taoist concept of "effortless doing."

As I stare across the table and Steve takes a bite of his hamburger, I see Pooh, my best dinner companion. Eeyore, the donkey, would depress me. He is a pessimist and complains incessantly. Eeyore can't just "be." Thank goodness I didn't marry an Eeyore. Looking around the cafeteria, I notice a lot of Eeyores. I nibble on my salad and I think about the other potential dinner companions from Pooh's crowd. How about Owl? Hoff says the owl is too wise for his own good. He over thinks everything and gets nothing done. He'd be eating dinner with me espousing and plotting and getting nowhere. I'd be frustrated with the owl. In my corporate days, we called it analysis paralysis. Dinner with Piglet would be the direct physical opposite of eating with Steve. Piglet is so small and cute, but he doesn't project confidence and is a worrier. The what-if scenarios would make me uptight. I'd rather focus on the facts than agonize over hypotheticals.

My mind is racing with this analogy. I know Steve would not be interested in the discussion, it's too abstract. So I smile at him. He seems content to be eating with me. What about Tigger? How would he be tonight? He's always bouncing and letting everyone know he goes the highest. He is amazed at himself. Well, Tigger is so impressed with his own abilities, he'd be bragging that he could fix the problem and tell the doctors a thing or two. Oh no: Maybe I have some Tigger in me! In the books, Tigger rarely accomplishes anything. I stay quiet.

Steve, my own Winnie-the-Pooh, knows how to help Gary. He says, "We'll just take one day at a time, one step at a time." It's so Winnie-the-Pooh simple. And so, we eat dinner, under the stars, by the candlelight and hold hands and look into each other's eyes.

It's been about an hour since surgery started. The doctor mentioned that if he could do it − whatever it is he's doing − laparoscopically, the procedure would take about two hours. If not, it could take longer. I'm optimistic we'll get a call within the next hour. Steve and I go back up to the room to wait.

I call my mom to update her and to see how she and Matt are doing. I'm not sure which of Pooh's friends describe my mom. She's her own breed, devoid of *wei wu wei*. I can tell instantly on the phone she is anxious because she starts yelling to me about Matt. He is not doing what she wants. He's stuck in the house with the "honey-do list." Since she is anxious about Gary, she just yells out her commands and expects Matt to drop everything. He needs to "put the newspaper away" or "bring the garbage down" or "bring up the laundry." He'd prefer her to bundle the list and do all the tasks at once instead of being in instant response mode. These are all things my mother used to be able to do herself. She is frustrated that she can't do them any longer. She feels bad that she is getting old and she drowns out her sorrows in anything pastry-like. She wants me to know we are out of bagels. Is she kidding me? Matt doesn't mind helping but he can't drive. He's 12. Normally, I'd be the Christopher Robin and mediate. I know I should take a deep breath, listen to the problem and help everyone find a solution. But tonight I am raw. Before I can stop myself I blurt out, "Stop stuffing your face and be my mother!"

Oh my God. I can't believe these words are coming out of my mouth. I have never spoken to her this way.

I continue, "I need you to listen to me! I need you to be supportive of me! I have spent 20 years working with you to give you tools to cope. I want you to know that as of tonight, I am done supporting you and teaching you coping mechanisms. You have all the tools you need. Now, I need you to implement them."

I am in shock. She is silent. I'm her only child and I have always been her rock. But, I am cracking. I feel awful, but I have no more capacity for this.

I whisper, "I have no more capacity. You'll have to find a way to be a support to me."

Finally, she breaks the silence. I'm expecting her to yell at me for being so inconsiderate but she calmly says, "I've never thought about things from your perspective."

More silence.

"I need you, Mom," I say, something I don't think I've ever admitted. "I know you can do it. I love you."

"I know," she says and hangs up.

I hang up the phone and Steve bursts out laughing. He repeats the refrain, "Stop stuffing your face and be my mother?"

I look at him, stunned.

"Wow," he says. "I've never heard you talk like that to her."

"I know."

Steve holds my hand and for a while we sit in silence. Nearly two hours have passed. No call from the doctor. Steve turns on a rerun of Law and Order. We watch a full hour episode. Another episode airs and we stare at the TV. Four hours have passed. What the hell is going on down there?

Finally, the phone rings, Gary is in recovery. The person tells us to come on down.

It is 1 a.m. and Gary is lying on the bed, asleep. He looks peaceful. Steve and I stand over him and just stare and stare and stare. Dr. Bennet, a tall, impressive man whose aura screams experience, and a young resident, too good-looking, with perfect teeth, wavy hair and you sense women fawn all over him, walk over to us. My exhaustion is replaced with the energy of skepticism.

"What took so long?" I blurt out.

Dr. Bennet states, "We could not do it laparoscopically. Gary had several adhesions. So we cut from his pelvis to about two inches above his belly button." The doctor lifts Gary's surgery gown and shows us his work. I am horrified at the cuts in my son. The incision goes straight past Gary's belly button, which looks like it's been cut out and sewn back in. It is disgusting. My baby has been cut to pieces. I feel sick inside. I can't imagine how long this recovery will be. Gary was just walking. He just was getting ready to go back to school! I manage to hold back my shock and let the doctor continue.

"I made four additional cuts for equipment." (I have no idea what this means. He points to puncture wounds.) "I took out the entire intestine and then replaced it back. I inserted a fabric to reduce the chance of having scar tissue. The good news is there is no Crohn's to be seen."

So this surgery had nothing to do with Crohn's, nothing to do with rice, and nothing to do with Gary's bladder? Then what was it for? My brain is working in overdrive. I am trying to think quickly to sort out the critical issues and focus. I know it is late and they probably want to go home. I don't care. Why are there four punctures in addition to the huge slice that runs from my son's pelvic bone and beyond? The incision is literally three times the size of my

Caesarian section incision. My C-section pulled out Gary, who was a 10-pound-3-ounce baby. What on earth did they have to take out and replace that was so big? And why? This is the pivotal issue. Like a surgeon with precision, I cut to it.

Looking at the resident smiling next to the doctor as if he were the winner of the suck-up contest to watch the surgery, I ask, "Who did this surgery?"

In the past, I wouldn't have asked about who did the surgery. But this is a teaching hospital. Did something happen during that first surgery that brought us back here? Dr. Bennet quickly responds "I did. The resident observed and helped with closing only. It took 45 minutes just to sew him back up."

I shudder at the thought of that.

"Why did he need this surgery? And what's that fabric you mentioned?"

"Gary had scar tissue from the first surgery. This resulted in multiple adhesions. I made sure to look for all of them and removed them. I like to use fabric," he continued, "because it helps prevent scar tissue."

This is the first explanation I am getting about "adhesions." Did they already know the adhesions were there when I was ranting about the rice? Is this why Dr. Hughes knew to send Gary to surgery right away? Did they just humor me with the roto-rooter? What a horrifying thought. I am furious. If I go into attack mode, I'll get mumbo jumbo and made to feel inferior because I do not have their training or technical knowledge. So I smile widely as I say, "So there was no damage from Crohn's," making sure to sound so pleased. I try to sound like a subservient female, someone who needs comforting, who the doctor can rescue with simple words. "So, Doctor, I am scared. How do I know that Gary will not have the same problem from this surgery?"

"Well, there can always be scar tissue. But I used the fabric." He repeats the words "scar tissue" and "fabric" again as if they are commonplace. He continues with, "I use it frequently."

Using my sweet voice, I ask, "What does this fabric do again?"

"It reduces the chance of scar tissue," he says with an authoritarian flair, a tone designed to give me comfort. It's a doctor voice – the firm low intonation that demonstrates he is in control and needs few words.

We are trained at GE to identify the root cause of a problem. I'll use my engineering protocol to figure this out. "Did they use it the first time?" I say, since, apparently, the first surgery caused the need for this surgery. I know this is the critical question, but I act pretty matter-of-fact so I don't get a defensive answer. I smile as I wait for his answer.

"I don't know," he says.

Action item for later: Find out if they used the fabric the first time and if not, why not. Determine if this is the root cause of the problem or if there might be something else. Verify that the second surgery does not change Gary's choice of maintenance using nutrition and not medications.

The doctor returns Gary's gown over the bandage. Steve and I return to the sixth floor and I see some familiar nurses' faces. I'm grateful to see that the male nurse, Jeff, is on duty and is getting the room ready. I'm exhausted and I know he is a pro at aftercare and managing the beeping machines. It will make Steve's and my stay here tonight a little more tolerable. As we wait for Gary to arrive, Jeff walks over to me and shakes my hand. In a daze, I hear him thank me.

"For what?"

"The letter you wrote to the hospital CEO made an impact. He read it to the staff. We all got recognition. I really appreciate what you did," he says.

I'd completely forgotten about the letter. I wrote it when Gary was being tutored and sent it out last week. Thank goodness I did that – before this happened – because I'm not feeling very grateful to be back here.

Gary is wheeled into the room. Jeff gets busy checking the monitors while someone else brings in a cot for Steve. We get ready for bed as Jeff tends to Gary. My mind is racing. Three weeks after his first surgery, when Gary started to feel ill, the pediatrician and everyone else said not to fret, he probably had a stomach bug. Forty-eight hours of continuous vomiting later – when all that came up was bile – I brought him to the E.R., where they took an X-ray. I don't think I heard a word about scar tissue or adhesions. In Hartford, with the U.G.I. study, no one said anything about adhesions. I convinced them to try the roto-rooter – which could never remove scar tissue! And all this time, it turns out that scar tissue is not uncommon after intestinal surgery.

I look over to Steve, who looks exhausted. I can't hold back my thoughts. "Honey," I say, "I wonder if the first doctor used this fabric."

Steve doesn't respond. He's already sleeping.

What You Can Do Now

1. Accept reality.

There is a "for worse." How we handle life's obstacles is how we make it "for better."

2. Look for the root cause of the problem.

The root cause is the issue that all others stem from. If you solve that one first, many of the others disappear. I make a list. I prioritize the biggest issues and attack those first. The challenge is staying focused. Many times side issues appear and they are easier to tackle. If someone keeps bringing up a side issue, I acknowledge them and thank them but reinforce I am working on other issues at the moment.

* * *

Chapter 15

My Son's Heart

The closed vertical blinds protect the hospital room from the intrusion of the bright morning sun. From my couch-bed, I sway a couple of panels and notice the sun's been up for a while. I put on my eyeglasses and shine enough light to see Gary's face. He looks peaceful. We must have overslept through the resident alarm clock. Perhaps they remembered not to flash on the overhead lights and to whisper. Both Steve and Gary are still sleeping. I know that Gary will mostly sleep for the next couple of days. He'll just want me here to give him some sips of ice and to call the nurses if the machines beep incessantly.

The days will move slowly. Like a train pulling out of its station, it will take a while for Gary to restart and get up to speed. I feel like a Porsche, at least in my mind. What if he has scar tissue from this surgery, too? What if he can't try nutritional therapy because of the second surgery? When will he be able to go back to school? If the school administrators thought it was dangerous to have him in the halls with the first incision, wait till they hear about this! Gary's whole middle was ripped open. There's no way he can play tennis. Maybe he should just drop the year. How do I tell him that? How do we get more information, rather than simply react to this crisis? It feels like we are on a path with no lights. Why do we have to live in the dark? Where is the light at the end of this tunnel?

I yank open the blinds. The burst of bright wakes Steve. Gary doesn't even stir. I get off of my couch and kiss Steve good morning. Then we both just stare at Gary. There's no point in us both staying here, so I send Steve home to buy the bagels (it will help reduce my mom's anxiety) and take Matt out to lunch. I'm sure Matt is miserable and my mom is probably in a massive funk. I'm sure she didn't sleep last night after I challenged her to "be my mother." Her mom was killed in a car accident when my mother was three. My mother was taken in by her grandmother, who had seven of her own children. My mother basically raised herself. It's the same parenting technique she used with me. My mom never got over the loss of her mother. She didn't have the capacity for my issues plus hers. I learned quickly to take care of myself.

Normally, I'd go home and spend hours consoling her, but this time I can't. Gary is eight hours post-op, so I'm staying put. It's Sunday, food shopping day, and we need to get some routine back. Who knows how long Gary will be here this time?

Steve washes up and kisses a sleeping Gary goodbye. I walk him to the elevator. As I stroll back to the room, I see the Indian mom pushing her son in a wheelchair. Her son looks slightly better but she looks noticeably worse. We wave to each other.

Back in Gary's room, a nurse attends to Gary. When she turns around, I notice it's Laura, the pudgy middle-aged, seen-it-all nurse, from the last time we were here. She's the one who said, "Remember, it's a blip," referring to Gary's life journey and the surgery.

"Some blip," I shout. My son is lying there with a morphine pump and I'm terrified this will happen again and again.

"I am so sorry," she says, like she means it.

"Blip?" I say again. I stare at her. She says nothing. I continue, "I think it's a blip, blip, *blooooop.*" I emphasize the last word like it's a train falling off a bridge and crashing. That other man said his kid had 15 surgeries. Fifteen surgeries on a girl of 19! I walk over and stand right in front of her, nose to nose. All of the restraint I exercised with not bombarding my husband and the doctors with questions is gone. She's an expert. I pound out the questions like she is my verbal punching bag.

"How could we not have known to watch for bile?" I don't wait for a response. "The scar is huge. What did they do in there?" I inch closer. "How much longer for this recovery?" Then I scream, "AND HOW LONG UNTIL WE'RE BACK IN HERE AGAIN?"

She doesn't flinch. She responds, calmly. "Randi, this will add three more weeks to his recovery. Trust me. I've seen this before. It's an extra three weeks."

I step back. Three weeks. It's not forever.

"How do you know?" I say.

"I've been around a long time," she says. She looks like it. She looks older than the first surgeon by two decades at least.

"What if it happens again?" I'm not sure I want to hear her answer.

"You can't focus on what might happen," she says. "You have to deal with your reality. At this point, it's an extra three weeks."

She looks at Gary and says to me, "He'll go home again. He'll recover again. He'll get the tutors again. And he'll go back to his life, again."

She doesn't say it but I suspect she means unlike some of the other kids on the floor. The Indian boy had a massive head trauma. He is not going back to his regular life.

"An extra three weeks?"

"Yes," she says.

I take a breath and take a seat on the chair by the desk.

"So, I should start my spa ritual again?" I say, forcing myself to laugh.

Gary must have been listening. He uncovers his face from the blanket. I want to wrap my arms around him. "Mom, I can handle three extra weeks," he mutters. "We know the drill. I'll be walking around the floor before you know it. Where's that thing with the blue ball?"

He's one step ahead of me, that boy. "What about the scar tissue?" I say to the nurse. "Won't it be worse this time because the incision is so much bigger?"

"Sometimes adhesions happen. But it doesn't mean they will happen again. You can spend your energy on what might happen but that is not going to help you help Gary recover."

Gary takes a hit from the morphine pump. Then he looks up at the nurse and mumbles, "Can you explain to my mom that this is just an extra sentence in my life story. When I'm 60, I'll just need to add a sentence: When I was 15, I had two operations and missed some of my sophomore year of high school." The nurse looks directly at me and I at her. I can't believe his perspective.

"He's right," the nurse says. "It's an extra sentence. Help him to not make it more."

I run over to hug my wise son, but he's already conked out again, without taking his first breath in the tube. I sit on the couch and stare out the window. Help him not make it more, I think to myself. The mountains-out-of-molehills lesson. I think of my mother-in-law. Steve's mom climbed every six-inch molehill with the drama of a Mount Everest summit. She passed away in 2008. I hate to say it but she evolved from a svelte, blonde, blue-eyed bombshell to the look of a beached whale in a 71-year life span. It was so sad. If she were alive today I'm sure she'd be on the phone with me continually looking for status updates on Gary's progress, so that she could worry more. She prided herself on this trait. She'd say that worry was how to show love.

"You only worry about people you care about," she'd say. In my marriage, it got to a point that even when things were fine, she looked for a problem, because that gave her a way to show her "love." When a problem appeared, even small stuff like fixing the car transmission, she'd use the refrain, "It's always something." I wished she'd help me figure out a solution and not just make never-ending phone calls for status updates. Even if we fixed the car, she'd call to see if the car needed another repair, because what if her son loses his job then we couldn't afford a new car? She was never happy because she lived in fear that something would go wrong. She was the living Piglet and Eeyore combination.

Instead of me enjoying wonderful memories of her, I recall an unhappy person whose doctors prescribed medications to help her deal with her ever-increasing list of ailments. She spent her days watching TV, munching on Hershey's chocolate bars and calling me for updates. Her weight crept up. She was prescribed cholesterol medication and diabetes medication. She ended up with anemia, restless leg syndrome, COPD and fibromyalgia, all conditions that required even more medication. No one ever prescribed that she change her behaviors. For example, she never ate a vegetable; she hated them since she was a kid. Medicare even paid over $1,000 for vitamin B shots twice a month. *Just eat your broccoli!* I wanted to tell her. Instead she took more than 20 pills a day. They generated so many side effects that she got sicker and sicker until she died. My heart broke for her and her family.

"Help him not make it more." Laura's words echo in my mind. The sun begins to warm me. In spite of his brief moments of lucidity earlier, I know Gary will sleep most of the day away. So, I spend the first 24 hours post-op, eating my "spa" cuisine, writing the day's events, taking my 4 p.m. power walk and at night going to the meditation room down the hall. There's a big, black massage chair in the center of a small room with no windows. Along the walls are bookshelves lined with inspirational books and lavender hand creams, which I generously spread up my arms and take a big whiff of. I dim the lights, gaze at the glow-in-the-dark stars on the ceiling and fill the room with Harry Conick Jr's jazz. The stars shine and I use the remote control to turn on the massage chair. The chair massages the back of my head and my calves at the same time. Plus, there is this rolling motion on my back. Oh my goodness, the chair is amazing. I feel my tight muscle knots disappearing. I can make the kneading motion as strong as I want. The CD remote also lets me play the same song over and over again.

I hope Harry doesn't mind singing repeatedly:

"Smile though your heart is aching
Smile even though it's breaking
When there are clouds in the sky, you'll get by
If you smile through your fear and sorrow
Smile and maybe tomorrow
You'll see the sun come shining through ... for you.
Light up your face with gladness
Hide every trace of sadness
Although a tear may be ever so near
That's the time you must keep on trying
Smile, what's the use of crying?
You'll find that life is still worthwhile
If you just smile."

I listen to the song so many times and feel so good from the massage, I walk out of the room glowing. The wise nurse is right. I will not make this more than it is.

The next morning, I hear the residents poking around. They're examining Gary's incision. They say he is progressing well. But, with almost back-to-back surgeries, and my journal from the last time, Gary's recovery seems slower to me. I guess it is because he really wasn't fully recovered from the first surgery. Gary hasn't blown into the tube yet to keep pneumonia at bay. He just seems to want to hit the morphine pump. A doctor stops by and says they have a little procedure that will help with Gary's recovery.

"Gary, we are going to insert a PICC line so that the antibiotics and nutrients can be easily absorbed by your body," he says with authority. "You will be able to watch the line go up through your arm and into the vein and pass directly in front of your heart on the monitors." They are starting to understand that Gary appreciates detail.

I would like more information, though. For example, what do they mean this is going up a vein to his heart to deliver the medications? I hate the idea of antibiotics to begin with and now they are sending the antibiotics directly into his heart? I hear someone mention the chance of infection from the PICC line and all the protocol stuff they are legally responsible to say. I do not think I sign any additional forms for the procedure; I guess I am on board at this point. I'm accepting the protocol. I add a dose of prayer to give me hope. Gary is hooked up to four antibiotics, plus morphine. I did not want Gary to take more drugs, but I'm not the one having the procedure. I don't question what PICC stands for, a sign to me of capitulation to the process. Look what I did with roto-rooter. I don't need to make this more than a sentence in his life story. I wait for Gary's reply.

He hasn't said much since the surgery, but musters up the strength for the critical question. "Does it hurt?"

"No it doesn't," the doctor says, adding, "We can give you some relaxants so you are less anxious during the procedure. You will be awake but you won't care."

"If it doesn't hurt, I want to be alert. I want to watch it," Gary says, suddenly fully awake, and with the excitement of a kid being told he'll be going to the World Series, not just watching it on TV.

"You can be in the room as well, Mom, and watch," the doctor says.

Oh joy. I hate operations. I hate blood. But how do I not watch this? After all, I go to all his ball games and talent shows. How do I say NO to this?

The attendant maneuvers Gary's bed and his contraptions to the elevator. We are off to the procedure room. Gary is alert, the most awake I've seen him since the surgery. The elevator seems to move at a normal pace today. The elevator doesn't even feel like a prison cell. I don't even want to escape. I'm traveling like this is now part of my life.

The procedure room seems dark to me. It is not meant to be dark, the operating lights overhead shine brightly, but the windowless room feels isolated. I have no sense of perspective of place. I could be in an underground tunnel or in a spaceship. It's like in the movies when the aliens take the captive to a room to do a procedure. The aliens all look alike, yet all seem unique in their role and the process. They work in unison and the captive stares out silently. I'm watching this like a movie, but I'm in it. Someone mentions again that there is a high risk of infection with the procedure. A nurse whisks a blue gown and cap on me. I wear a face mask as well. There are monitors everywhere and nearby waits a table with a blue cloth over it. Is that where they are going to lie Gary down? No. A nurse pushes Gary's bed to the other side of the room, next to another bed. Gary, who just had a second surgery, lifts his body up as the nurses pull the blanket from one bed to the other.

A nurse comes by my side and lifts the blue tablecloth on what I thought was a bed. Underneath, I see the scalpel and surgical equipment. I've never been this close to this stuff. It's so shiny and sharp. My knees wobble. I ask for a chair.

I can't even watch medical shows on TV without closing my eyes and now I am sitting here hearing a doctor say, "Gary, I'll make the incision here." He points to Gary's upper arm. He holds up a long, slender, small, flexible tube. "The tube will travel in your large vein and pass by your neck and go toward your heart. Do you want something to help you relax?"

Gary responds, "No."

I want something to relax! Ask me!

The doctor continues talking to Gary, "OK, I'll tell you every step in the process."

"Great!"

The doctor asks for a scalpel, just like on TV. The nurse hands it to him. The doctor leans in toward Gary. He makes a cut. I look away from the doctor's hand and focus on Gary's face. Gary watches the knife open his skin. I hear the doctor and Gary talking, but I feel queasy. The only thing keeping me from fainting is Gary's excitement. Gary is looking at the monitors and giving a play-by-play of the position of the wire.

I hear him say, "I see my veins." Pretty soon, I hear him exclaim, "That's my heart. It's right there."

My son's heart.

Moments later, the doctor confirms the procedure is complete. He seems to be securing the catheter and mentions it should not move out of the insertion site on Gary's arm. It looks like a sterile dressing is placed on it to protect it from infection. Gary turns to me and says, "This is better than school, Mom. They don't teach this stuff there!" He says it from his heart, figuratively and literally.

"They certainly don't, honey."

I'd rather he be in biology class.

What You Can Do Now

---

1. Talk to the nurses.

They are the front line. They have perspective. They work with many doctors and know the results of surgery. At first, I tried taking out my frustration on the nurse, but luckily she did not get defensive. She knew she was not the problem; she was part of the solution. Nurses know how long recovery takes, the problems to be expected and lessons learned from other cases.

2. Worry doesn't accomplish anything.

After the second surgery, I worried about a third and fourth. But worrying about what might happen takes away energy from fixing what has already happened.

3. The song is right.

As Harry Connick Jr. sings, smile though your heart is aching.

* * *

Chapter 16
Figuring the Fail Rate

Back in the room, I Google PICC line on my laptop while Gary rests. Too much medical information has scared me in the past so I know this can be dangerous. When Steve had nodules on his thyroid, I became convinced he was going to die of cancer because of what I read on the Internet. I swore off medical Internet searches. But this seems like a benign procedure, no pain, quick and, for Gary, even fun. So, I type PICC line. In 0.11 seconds I have over 200,000 results. I click on the second option – What is a PICC line and why do I need it. I love Google! I skim the website and my first question is answered. PICC stands for Peripherally Inserted Central Catheter. Apparently, a PICC line terminates right near the heart to allow for treatment that you can't get from standard I.V. access. The PICC line can stay in place for a much longer duration than other central or periphery access devices[8], which I guess means a regular I.V.

A PICC line is used for prolonged I.V. antibiotic treatment and TPN nutrition. Does this mean they are preparing him for an even longer stay? Not sure what TPN stands for, but anything that nourishes him should be good. He is skin and bones. I click the section about risks of the PICC line. Maybe I should have read this beforehand; I would have had more questions for the doctors. Apparently, air bubbles may enter the blood vessel during insertion of a PICC and the patient's blood pressure can decrease. I had no idea about nerve injury or irritation or paralysis[9] during catheter insertion either! Gary didn't complain of any shooting type of pain down his arm, numbness, or tingling. He was smiling when they finished, so I guess that's a good sign. I hope there isn't a next time, but if there is, I'll at least ask about the number of times the doctor has completed the procedure and his record of results. Lesson learned: Experience is key for this procedure. According to the site, Gary's not out of the clear just yet. He still has risks of infection and phlebitis (an inflammation of the vein where the catheter is inserted). I need to watch for redness in two places now, by his belly incision and on his arm.

Gary sleeps soundly again the second day. He doesn't say much. He's not breathing in the tube like last time. I try to give it to him, but he is totally exhausted. Everyone says he is progressing as expected. I check for redness myself and don't see any spreading. To calm my nerves, I write a little, I take my power walk. I eat a salad for dinner and take a hot bath before sleeping on the couch at night.

On day three, Gary coughs, a deep cough. He sounds terrible. I reach under my pillow for my glasses and rush outside to tell the residents. I don't care about my frizzed-out hair, my morning breath or being seen in my husband's T-shirt in the hospital hall.

"Gary is coughing. You guys did such a great job this morning not disturbing us that Gary didn't wake up. But he's coughing now and his lungs sound awful," I say. I sound as scared as I must look. Is this the start of pneumonia? A couple of residents immediately return to the room. Gary coughs for them. It's a loose gurgling cough. They check his lungs. I'm scared sick. I shouldn't have let him sleep so much yesterday. I should have started the ball log. One of the beeping machines goes off. I feel like it's only a preliminary buzzer to whatever the next real distress is. Gary must sense my concern. He finally answers the question I've been avoiding asking the past two days.

Gary suppresses a cough and then he says, "Mom, I have no pain. I feel great, just some surgery pain."

The residents whisper to each other. One of the residents says Gary needs to use the ball contraption. The antibiotics should help kill any infections. Gary coughs again. *Oy*. I look at the pumps and the bags of fluids. They are filling him up with four types of high dose antibiotics. I hate that stuff. It's probably what can help prevent pneumonia, but I still ask, "Does he really need all four of them?"

"Mrs. Oster, he needs the antibiotics to fight infection. He had major surgery. It will only be for a few days," a young resident replies.

The surgeon said there was no inflammation and no Crohn's. Maybe a couple of days of high-dose antibiotics won't hurt. Once Gary gets home, I'll put him on a probiotic. I don't recall anyone in the hospital ever even mentioning them to me. When I asked, they said it couldn't hurt.

The residents leave and before Gary falls back asleep I hand him a piece of paper, a pen and the ball contraption. He knows exactly what he has to do. Last time he was walking by Day Two. Not this time. It's Day Three and he still needs to sit up on the side of the bed. The nurse said three extra weeks. Well, this certainly is a slow start.

After my morning routine of showering and purchasing oatmeal from the cafeteria, I watch Gary sleep and pull out my laptop to write. I never expected to be back here, at least not so soon. As my fingers race on the keyboard, Dr. Carroll, the first surgeon from three weeks ago, knocks on the door. I look up and wave him in. Gary perks up. He's told me repeatedly he is so grateful to Dr. Carroll for stopping the peeing pain. To Gary, he is a miracle-worker.

Dr. Carroll comes in and investigates Gary's multiple scars. Gary has an upside down "T" on his belly with seven smaller incisions from both surgeries. It looks like a mess to me. The doctor focuses primarily on the horizontal scar below the belly button. That one is his. It is still red and raised. Even if Gary's bare skin grows hair, I don't see how the scar won't show through. I am concerned Gary will feel self-conscious in a bathing suit. I don't say anything, but Dr. Carroll must suspect it is on Gary's mind as well.

He appeals to Gary's macho side as he examines Gary's belly. "You know, the girls will dig the scar."

"Really?"

"Yeah. They will want to touch it," Dr. Carroll says.

"Awesome."

So, the scars are cool. My obsession about them is probably from a bikini-wearing female's perspective, not a hormone raging teenage boy's.

As Dr. Carroll examines Gary's belly, I need to determine if Dr. Carroll used the fabric. In GE, I was trained to find the root cause of a problem. If you fix it, many other subsequent issues may fade away. I think the lack of fabric may be the root cause of the need for the second surgery. The fabric supposedly reduces scar tissue. I did not tell Gary about the fabric and how maybe the second surgery could have been avoided. How maybe if it had been used he'd be back in school today, he'd be getting stronger for tennis, he'd not be in pain from recovering from a second surgery.

I take a deep breath. Stay calm to gain control, I remind myself. I don't want to make Dr. Carroll defensive. Then it will be harder to get the answer about the fabric. I need to seem friendly. I ask the hard question about the fabric, sounding as innocent as possible.

"Dr. Carroll, it's nice for you to have stopped by to see Gary." I smile warmly.

"The first incision is healing nicely," Dr. Carroll reports to me.

"That is great to hear. Gary has no pain any longer when urinating. Thanks so much," I say and he smiles back.

I continue with a smile, "Dr. Carroll, I understand that Gary had adhesions from the first surgery and this caused the blockage. Dr. Bennet said he used this special film or fabric to help prevent new adhesions from this surgery."

"Oh, yes. I am very familiar with the film. I was one of the doctors who was on the research team to test its viability. I remember the study well. In the end, we found it inconclusive."

"Did you use the fabric?" I ask softly.

"I am not sure if I used it because Gary's area was small."

"Doctor, I'd like to know. Actually it is better news for us if you did not use the fabric. It might explain why this might have happened. Since it was used the second time, at least a new step was taken to prevent it from happening again." I feel like I am talking to a child, trying to make him not feel bad about his choice to not use the fabric and wanting him to tell me the truth.

"I understand," he says. "I have to check to see if I used the fabric. I'll get back to you." Dr. Carroll leaves the room.

Gary asks me a couple of questions about his operation. I explain how this time Dr. Bennet used a fabric that reduces the chances of scar tissue. I don't know if Dr. Carroll used it. If not, I feel like he put Gary on an express train to the low road. Gary interrupts me. "Mom, being mad at the doctor won't change anything." He says this from the high-road perspective. Maybe my teachable moments have sunk in too well. But, this is beyond a brother squabble over a toy truck when I tell Gary to take the high road and let his little brother play first. I think we are allowed to be angry if the doctor could have minimized the chances of a need for a second surgery. I'm heading directly for the low road myself.

Steve unexpectedly pops in. He knew we'd need a visitor! It's been three days since the surgery. He is working from his Connecticut office today. It's lunchtime. He kisses Gary hello and Gary tells us to take our time and eat in the cafeteria. I think Gary wants me and my negative energy out of the room. Steve holds my hand as we walk to the elevator. It does nothing to calm me down but I stay quiet. I don't know who is around us and my cynicism is sky high. Not the best formula for insuring Gary gets the best care.

Steve and I rush downstairs for a quick bite. Midweek lunch is a sharp contrast to Saturday night dining in this place. Now, it's bustling. As expected, all of the birds still flock together. We walk past the tables of doctors and sit at a table for two. I munch on my salad and tell Steve how Dr. Carroll did not remember if he used the fabric. I can't believe it; you'd think he'd know. He said he was familiar with it but couldn't commit an answer? Wouldn't you know what materials you used in an operation? I remember working on aircraft instrumentation and as engineers we were neurotic over the least little design change of a flange. The slightest change could affect engine performance. Planes could crash! As I talk to Steve, my hands are flailing as I describe the precision required for jet engines. How do you not know if you used the fabric? I am definitely not in a Pooh state. I see Dr. Carroll leaving his flock and coming toward us. Deep down, I am hoping he says he did not use the fabric. This way, maybe this time, Gary won't get adhesions. I anxiously look up at Dr. Carroll. I don't even ask the question again.

He smiles and says, "No fabric."

"Thank you. That is great news." I beam with joy.

"No problem." Dr. Carroll returns to his flock.

I look at Steve. I'm relieved, yet torn. I'm grateful that there's no more peeing pain, and aghast that he didn't remember Gary's procedure, and perplexed over why he wouldn't have used the fabric. Maybe this time the fabric will reduce the chance of us being back here in three weeks, again. Dr. Bennet seems to think so. At least Steve and I quickly finish lunch to tell Gary the news. Gary seems relieved. He takes a deep breath in the ball contraption, I think to show off to his dad. Steve high-fives Gary before leaving for work. With things looking up, I continue writing. I find it easier to focus when things are positive.

Gary falls asleep. I look around the room. There are significantly fewer flowers, stuffed animals and cards this time in his hospital room. I told most people to stay home and not to send another batch of goodies. We know we are loved from the outpouring the first time. The kids from the Hebrew school did a nice job of sending another batch of cards. But I hope this doesn't become a monthly project for them. I pray Dr. Bennet is right about the fabric and I realize I was wrong about kids without decorations in the room. It doesn't mean their families are not connected to the community. It just may mean that the child is a frequent flier. I have to remember to always send something.

I haven't been outside in days. It looks cold and gray out there. As Gary sleeps, I type away in the warm room. I never expected so much material – I wish I didn't have so much material! I can get my clients' e-mails on my laptop and call in for messages and my business partner, Reena, is handling any appointments I can't make. Thank goodness for Reena. Just as I am thinking of her, I hear a knock on the door. I get up to open it and a frozen-looking Reena is standing in the hall. I tell her we should head down to the cafeteria for some hot tea. She doesn't say it, but I know she is sad to see me back here so soon. Her daughter had back-to-back surgeries just a year ago. She too had to train the residents to let her daughter sleep. She understands hospitals are not a quiet place and it's claustrophobic to spend hour after hour, day after day, week after week in a 10-by-20 room.

I remember hearing about her tribulations, but I couldn't relate. I went to visit her and her daughter in Bridgeport Hospital after the first surgery, but can't remember if I sent anything the second time. I remember Reena going to three different children's hospitals before she settled on one in Pennsylvania for the second surgery. She did a lot more homework than I did. So far, so good for her daughter. She was careful about picking a surgeon and even a support team. I look at Reena, a very successful long-term-care specialist. She is my business partner and is an excellent reader of people. It's a critical skill in selling. I don't want to come across to her as unsure of myself. Even though I am my own boss, I still have trepidations about appearing weak at work. I don't want to feel like I made a mistake by taking Gary to this hospital. Because then maybe I am a bad mother. Reena's business is significantly bigger than mine, making her even busier than I am. Yet she still did the research when it came to her child's surgery. I used the "trust" approach. As I ramble about the good news about the second surgeon using the fabric and the fact that the first surgeon didn't, I know I am rationalizing. This happens frequently in sales. When a client purchases a product, they will tell their friends about it and then, to convince themselves they did the right thing, they will refer the agent. Think of the many times people say, "I have the best real-estate agent!" Or financial planner, or lawyer or doctor or long-term-care specialist? When their friends use the same service, it legitimizes their original decision. Look at how Bernie Madoff took advantage of this human character trait.

I practically brag about the hospital and the second surgeon. "Look, Gary had adhesions, which is a risk of surgery, any surgery. But this time the doctor used this special fabric which reduces the chance of adhesions."

I see the obvious question start to form on her lips but I don't even let her ask it.

"The first doctor was involved in the research of the fabric and he felt the results of the benefits were inconclusive. I'm glad to know he didn't use it. Because now that it was used maybe the results will be different," I say, trying to convince her – and myself – that I didn't do wrong by my son.

Reena doesn't ask me any questions. I ramble on and on about how this time it should be different. I let her know it is a blip… just an additional three weeks… he'll be back to school… he'll play tennis again… it's a sentence in Gary's life story. She takes a sip of tea. She smiles as I excitedly tell her we are almost out of the woods. I can finally see the light.

I tell her I know this machine. I know the checkout girl in the cafeteria. I know the woman who cleans the room. I know the day nurse, the night nurse, the PCAs, the attendants, even the sitter for the suicide person. I know my neighbors and even the woman on Wednesday who brings the dog to the rooms for pet therapy. It is just like when I am at Trader Joe's grocery store and I run into people in the aisles and we stop and chat. I feel like I am part of a community. Like in my college days, when I had friends all over campus and I'd run into them in the dining hall. Just like in GE, I loved eating in the cafeteria and joining a table of coworkers and we'd laugh the hour away. It makes me feel like I'm part of something. It didn't take long for me to develop that here as well. Originally, I didn't want to be part of this community, but I like the people. I like the nurses. I like that the residents listen. I like that I learned the rhythm of this place. I like that I trusted the doctors with the PICC line. There are processes here that handle thousands of patients. Believing in the system is a positive energy. And that, I truly believe, helps Gary. The doctors have protocol and I have prayer. I tell Reena all this. By the time I am done espousing how wonderful the hospital is, I think she actually believes me.

I feel a tap on my shoulder. I turn around and I can't believe my eyes. It is Cathy, the mother of two, one with cerebral palsy who had an emergency bowel surgery and the other with autism. I am bumping into a friend here. Just like at Trader Joe's. She must be back for a routine check-up.

"Great to see you!" I say. I am excited to introduce her to Reena. I feel popular and connected.

"You too," she says. "Why are you here?"

I ooze breeziness as I say, "Oh, Gary had some complications from the first surgery. He had adhesions. They did an emergency second surgery the other night. He is doing much better now."

Her face changes, the smile evaporating. "My son too," she says. "He's been here about four days already."

"Wait," I say. "He had surgery. Again. Too?"

"Yes. Adhesions."

This can't be. I gulp my tea. I try to compose myself. Here I am bragging to Reena about this place, the people, the processes, and Cathy's son is back with the same complication as Gary. I cut to the key question, "Wasn't Dr. Carroll your first surgeon?"

"Yes, Dr. Carroll."

I feel sick to my stomach as the reality sinks in. Two surgeries by the same doctor, within one day of each other, and both children are back in the operating room within three weeks due to the same complication? Dread overcomes me. I grab onto the table with both hands. I see Cathy's other son running around the cafeteria, seeming very agitated. Cathy ignores him and stares at me. I cannot believe we are both back.

"Where is your son?" I ask.

"In a room on the other side of the hall from where Gary was after the first surgery," she says.

"We're on opposite sides of the floor. Luckily we bumped into each other here. Otherwise I'd have no idea you were back," I respond. They only have one floor for non-cancer post-op surgery for kids, and they put us at opposite ends. Can our room location be intentional? I hope not. I am speechless. Cathy sits down at our table. Her face is drawn white. Finally, she breaks the silence, changing the subject. "Randi, watch out if your insurance company has a limit. Mine does and we hit it."

Here is a new issue. I haven't a clue if we have a limit. No one mentioned a limit when Steve checked about our coverage. Is it because we don't have one or it didn't apply? I want to get to the root cause of the surgery first, before I worry about a financial catastrophe. Part of my training is to focus on critical issues and not get side-tracked.

"Did they use the fabric, the first time?" I say.

"What fabric," she asks.

"To prevent adhesions," I respond, like this is a solution that everyone should know about.

"I don't know," she says.

"Well Dr. Carroll didn't use it with Gary's first surgery. But Dr. Bennet did with the second surgery, so hopefully this won't happen again," I say, trying to convince myself as well. After all, I'm sure the goal here is wellness, not repeat procedures, right?

"I have to find out about this fabric," Cathy says, exasperated.

She grabs her other son and heads to the elevator.

"I'm in room 617," I say. "Let's talk later tonight. I know we'll both be here."

Reena walks over and gives me a hug, which is exactly what I need. I feel like I've been sucker-punched by this place. Cathy's son is back with the same complication? Limits on insurance? I stand limp in Reena's embrace. When she heads home I feel like my contact with the outside world leaves with her. I am stuck here in an alien spaceship.

I'll never know this for sure, but maybe the sad faces of the nurses when Gary returned to the hospital were due partly because they knew they had two repeat patients. If I hadn't bumped into Cathy in the cafeteria I would have never known both boys had the same complication. (Or in statistical lingo, the same outcome.) If it wasn't for me making friends with Cathy the first time, we would not have recognized each other the second time. Like most parents in the hospital, most of our days are spent in the room. I can count the minutes per day I leave Gary's side. The chance of meeting Cathy during this stay was really remote.

As I walk the corridors, my GE quality training rushes back to me. Before I left GE, I completed several Six Sigma projects. Six Sigma is a process improvement methodology designed to eliminate mistakes. Jack Welch, our CEO at the time, required every employee to strive to operate at the highest level of performance. A Six Sigma process is one in which 99.99966 percent of the products manufactured are free of defects. Six Sigma is all about improving processes to eliminate defects. It is an incredibly high standard: only 3.4 defects per one million parts. Many institutions operate at levels well below Six Sigma. A level of three sigma or lower is common, because the price of near perfection could raise the price of the product astronomically. Some things are not worth the effort to take them to the Six Sigma level (99.99966 percent defect-free). No one cares if 1 out of 100 matches (99 percent quality) breaks when lighting the barbecue. But everyone would like to be assured that the flow valve on the propane tank does not leak 1 percent of the time, causing an explosion when the match does ignite.[10] When operating at three sigma correlates to life and death, the negative consequences become clear. From my aircraft days, a three sigma is equivalent to two plane crashes per year at O'Hare International Airport. Unacceptable. And at three sigma, 20,000 wrong prescriptions per year are written. Also unacceptable, right? In health care, running at a 3.8 sigma, or 98.9 percent error-free rate, there are 5,000 defective surgical operations performed every week out of a million. By implementing and achieving a Six Sigma defect rate, 99.99966 percent, there would be 1.7 defective surgical operations every week out of a million.

I loved the quality programs at GE, more so than many of my colleagues did, because they fit my personality in that they're process-oriented. They're statistics heavy. But at their core, I loved the message: ***Don't blame people for the mistakes. Improve the process and the employees will perform better.*** Employees won't need to find a scapegoat in the organization to blame. They will develop a culture of teamwork to identify the root cause of a problem, fix it and move forward. I think Jack liked it because when the employees improved the process, we eliminated waste, we improved client satisfaction and we increased the bottom line. Whatever the motivation for implementing the Six Sigma program, it worked. We didn't sell on our sigma level, our customers just knew we delivered a consistent high-quality product.

Certainly, Gary's outcome and Cathy's son's outcome is not desirable, in terms of patient care, anyway. In GE, I bet I could get corporate funding for a Six Sigma study of this surgical process. But, I am no longer there.

I can't believe how easily the Six Sigma basics came back to me. Basically they come down to this: Figure out the problem and figure out a plan to fix it. Then fix it. Each Six Sigma project within

GE followed a defined sequence of steps, typically with goals such as improved quality or financial targets, like cost reduction or profit increase. I still remember the mnemonic for the steps: DMAIC. I think it is permanently logged into my brain. Each letter of the mnemonic is a distinct phase in the project.

1. Define   Define the problem and the project goals.

2. Measure Measure the current process and collect relevant data.

3. Analyze Analyze the data to investigate and verify cause-and-effect relationships. Seek out root cause of the defect under investigation.

4. Improve Improve or optimize the current process based upon data analysis. Set up pilot runs to establish process capability.

5. Control Control the future. State process to ensure that any deviations from target are corrected before they result in defects.

I wonder what sigma this place is operating at? It would be a pretty simple computation to figure out the number of defects over the total population. Take the operation that Gary had, for example. I'm guessing they do not think of Gary's result of the first surgery as a defect. But isn't it? In GE, a defect is defined as failure to deliver what the customer wants.[11] Certainly, Gary did not want a second surgery within the month. I wonder how they measure success? Or whether they do? The total population in this example has to be small. It's not like they do thousands of operations of this type each day. There aren't that many beds in this place. Walking through the halls, I go through the steps I would use to determine what's going on here.

1. Define the problem: Repeat surgeries due to adhesions. Goal: Reduce the chance of adhesions.

2. Measure: Collect data. I know of two surgeries in the last three weeks. How many surgeries are done a month? How many repeat visitors?

I can't start analyzing the data until I get the facts. As I approach Gary's room, I am thinking about my data collection plan and running some numbers in my head. How many surgeries like the one Gary and Andy had are done each month? Let's say it is a low number, like 10 a month. Assume that two go bad. That's a 20 percent fail rate. Even if the hospital did 20 a month and two went bad then it is still a 10 percent fail rate. When the nurse comes into Gary's room, my GE quality hat is on and I'm in Measure mode. I must sound like a crazy person, pounding out question after question, trying to get her to tell me how many procedures like the one Gary had a doctor typically does in a month, and the number of times she's seen the patients return so quickly. She scurries out of there, explaining that she must attend to another beeping machine. At GE, we embraced the data. But this environment is different. This is futile; she's never going to answer my questions. Even if she knows, she's not telling! Maybe the medical system has been burned by so many malpractice cases that the hospital feels the need to protect itself. Transparency is perceived as a problem, because the customers might sue. This is the exact opposite of using data to analyze the root cause and improve the system. I know that I am not going to blame her or the doctors. They helped my son, I know that. They are following current protocol. But the process is flawed!

The more I realize that I am not going to get the facts, the more frustrated I feel. I rove the floor chasing down nurses, demanding to know how many repeat patients have surgery due to adhesions. But no one will tell me. I am a bit hysterical. How many more times will Gary or another patient be back here with the same problem? In my state of mind this is becoming a horror movie. I flash back to "Rosemary's Baby." Once you are in, there is no escaping. Gary is tethered to the pumping machine contraption, with a tube snaking through his body and into his heart. He can't just pull it out and leave. I am obligated to have the same people who I think caused this problem, solve this problem.

And they are not forthcoming with information.

I walk the floor like a caged animal. I exhaust myself and return to Gary's room for some water. Just as I sit down, the child-life coordinator enters. Someone must have called for her to calm me down. Hospital protocol. She listened to both Gary and me after the first surgery. She is a good listener, but I fear that anything I say will be repeated to the people driving the protocol train. I have no privacy. She is not my friend. I feel like there is a conspiracy again. Still, I try to tell her my observations. After listening to my frustration with finding out about two repeat patients, she politely gets up and leaves. That's it. No resolutions. No promises. No hug.

How come there is no star rating for hospitals, like hotels? Why am I in the dark about overall performance? It's hard for me to trust anything right now. I'm waiting for the entourage to arrive again. When I was upset with Dr. Stark, because she did not call me for approval on a medication, she popped, like magic, into the room with three men. I go over to Gary and hold his hand and wait for the protocol machine to kick in, again. I am guessing the entourage will be here soon.

Gary looks up at me. He's so thin and so pale. He picks up on my energy and he hears me seething. He says, "Mom, Dr. Carroll solved my first problem. Dr. Bennet solved the second. Remember this is just one sentence of my life story." Even in my frazzled state I can see the man he'll become: calm, rational and a lemonade maker, just like his dad.

I sit and wait. Within minutes, there is a knock on the door. It's Dr. Bennet, without any back-up support. I like his approach. It exudes confidence. He smiles at Gary. He checks out Gary's belly and comes over to me on the couch. He does not sit down.

He says, "Gary is doing great. I want you to know that I used the fabric." I don't say anything. "They can't use the fabric if there is infection." He must be referring to the first surgery. It's almost as if he is stating a reason Dr. Carroll did not use the fabric. When Dr. Carroll eventually recalled that he hadn't used it he said it was because he did the research on the fabric and did not find it conclusive, plus the area was small. He never said anything about infection limiting his ability to use the fabric. I suspect the cover-up is starting. But there's no reason to start casting blame. So, I focus on data.

"Dr. Bennet, approximately how many intestinal surgeries per month are done here?" I say.

He looks up at me and says, without any doubt, "Five."

I am thrilled he is willing to give me an answer. But this is a lot fewer than I'd imagined. That means at least two out of five within a four-week period went bad. That is 40 percent.

I state the statistics. "So, two out of five went bad last month. That is 40 percent fail rate."

I know this sounds blunt but this is my GE experience talking. I am trained to face the facts, to look at the numbers, find the root cause and fix the problem. I am trained not to blame the person, but to improve the process. If the process is flawed, it doesn't matter who is working on the project, they will fail. Dr. Bennet's disposition changes. He says, "You can't do statistics on this type of procedure." He pastes on a smile and walks out of the room. He just walks out. I can't believe this. I take a deep breath. I guess I was too direct with him. I am used to engineers. We work as a team. We look at the numbers and figure out how to improve them. My failure rate analysis lacked emotion because I looked at the outcome of each surgery as if operated on a widget. He is looking at each case as a person. He is hearing me say the surgery fails the patient 40 percent of the time. That means he fails a human and a family. That must be painful for a doctor to hear. I know that doctors care about their patients. But looking at each situation individually prevents a person from seeing patterns. Quality is about removing deviation from the process. It's not personal.

The culture of the hospital is too different from GE. I can't change the hospital culture. Fighting the system will only weaken me. I have to find another way. I take another deep breath and look at Gary, who seems confused that the doctor stormed out.

"Know what? We can't change the wind, but we can change the direction of the sails," I tell Gary. I know he has heard me say this expression over and over again. Normally he rolls his eyes. No eye roll this time, though. Gary's sailing experience taught him if he wants the boat to speed up, he has to move the sails to take advantage of the wind. If a storm unexpectedly hits, he needs to change the sails to fly away. He can't just complain if there's too much wind, or if the wind is blowing in the wrong direction. He knows he has to adjust. So do I. Before I can help figure out how to improve this place, I've got to get Gary out of here.

I walk down the hall. I feel the stares from the nurses at the station. I feel like their eyes are following my every move. I am not going to sue. I am not going to do anything but try to help get Gary better. But I do not tell them this. I'll just continue to write down every interaction I have for a story to help other families cope. To help change the protocol. I know our story is not unique from a process perspective. Maybe even the medical community will gain a deeper understanding of the patient's viewpoint. As I approach Cathy's room, I feel as if I am adjusting my sails.

I pop my head into Andy's room and Cathy is in caged-animal mode. Before I say hello, she tells me she called the patient representative line to turn in Dr. Carroll. She says her husband looked up the effectiveness of the fabric on the Internet and discovered it is 80 percent. She screams, "So why wouldn't you just use it?" I nod to her, but I decide not to go there. I could easily add fuel to her fire. I could start bitching about this place again but I know nothing productive would come of it. So instead, I tell her about my book idea, about how our experience might help improve the plight for other moms and dads and kids.

She says, "It's better than a lawsuit. They are too prepared for that."

Her phone keeps ringing. She lets me know she is getting her son a new doctor and plans to get her son out of the hospital in time for Thanksgiving, tomorrow. This time, she writes her e-mail address down and says we'll keep in touch.

I hug her and say, "I hope we both get our kids off this train, soon."

She looks up at me. "I love that analogy. This is some trip."

What You Can Do Now

1. Read.

The doctors will only answer the questions you ask. Yes, the Internet can bombard you with information but it also helps you get a sense of critical issues. Some information on the Internet scared me, but at least I could be proactive with questions for the doctor.

2. Try not to make the doctor or any health care worker defensive.

They are doing their best. If they feel attacked they will close down. To sound less threatening when trying to obtain information, sandwich your concern between two positive statements. For example, "Gary seems to be doing better. By the way did you use the fabric? The pain is totally gone." By sounding positive and acknowledging that their effort is appreciated, you'll have a better chance at getting information.

3. If something goes wrong, stay calm.

They have processes built in for protecting themselves from lawsuits. Threatening will not bring you answers to your questions nor better care for your loved one. Instead, write down what happened. Record your understanding of the situation. Record their responses. Ask to speak with the patient advocate. Get the hospital to tell you what options you have. Wait to see if the "mistake" is really as bad as you suspect. If it is not too bad, tell them you expect it rectified to your expectations, and if not you'll be telling your friends on Facebook about the care received. If it truly is bad, get a lawyer.

* * *

Chapter 17
Giving Thanks

I wish I were home, especially today. Normally, the Wednesday before Thanksgiving, I buy the turkey, make fresh cranberry sauce with cinnamon and orange rinds, sauté onions for mushroom stuffing, and make fresh green beans with lemon and garlic. I set the table, with our good china, in the dining room for the family feast. Thanksgiving is my favorite holiday. It is about family. I love it. Instead, today, I am here writing down my operational observations.

There seems to be an even bigger push today than on Fridays to release patients. You have to be really sick to spend Thanksgiving in the hospital. For those who remain for the holiday, "Happy Thanksgiving" is a cruel refrain. It, appropriately, is not said to me by the workers. I tell Steve not to visit tomorrow. Traffic probably will be a nightmare and Matt deserves to have a traditional Thanksgiving at home. Steve agrees to stay home and cook our favorite family fixings for my mom and Matt. I recite the recipes over the phone. At this point, four days post-op, Gary has no cramps, just incision pain. He walks fairly steadily. He can make it around the entire floor. I've taken him on two trips so far today. When he is not increasing his endurance, he spends his day on his iPod, updating his Facebook friends. It is heartwarming and wrenching for me to read his updates. Over 600 "friends" instantly hear about his pain level, the huge scar, his first walk, and the number of times he's seen the "*Lord of the Rings*" trilogy. His friends from the Crohn's camp and "healthy" friends comment about his ordeal and post supportive messages. The Crohn's kids share their stories too. It's an open forum of the two worlds he's brought together. The "healthy" kids and Crohn's kids ask questions and Gary answers them for everybody to read.

I write, power walk, take a bath and check my e-mails and Facebook before bed. I force myself not to be sad that we will be spending Thanksgiving in the hospital. While I've been avoiding mentioning the holiday, I see on my laptop that Gary updates his Facebook status to wish everyone a "Happy Thanksgiving!" Within minutes, over 50 kids like his status. I love Facebook. I go to bed smiling.

Thanksgiving morning is just like any other in the hospital. As Gary waits for the "poop" to be released, he directs me to do push-ups in the room so I'll stay strong. Just as I am ready to collapse from his commands for "one more" the phone rings. It is Dan, Gary's high school buddy who is working with him to raise the money for the water pump in South Africa. Gary's eyes light up as he listens. All I hear is him saying, "No way," over and over again. I scream out, "What is it?" But he flails his hand telling me to basically shut up. He exclaims, "I can't believe it. Keep me posted!" He hangs up the phone.

I've not seen him this happy in what feels like forever.

"Mom, you are not going to believe this. Dan got an e-mail from Dana who has a potential donor for H2Africa for $90,000 to put in the water wells throughout the country!"

He is right, I can't believe it. Even in the hospital, Gary's been e-mailing Dan, his co-chair for the high school club – which the kids named H2Africa – about fundraising. This is amazing. I probe and it sounds like a long-shot, but I don't burst his bubble with reality. The thought of helping the people in Africa, instantly, puts the Thanksgiving back in the room. Gary is so excited that whenever a nurse comes in to check a monitor he tells him or her about the kids in Africa. How their moms walk four miles a day for water. How they live in houses smaller than his hospital room. How they don't have electricity for a DVD, or a shower in their room.

Gary's lunch tray is brought in and it's filled with turkey, stuffing, cranberry sauce and green beans. "This is amazing," Gary says, smiling broadly as he devours the meal. He is so happy with the news, cafeteria turkey never tasted so good! I look out the window, up at the sky and whisper thank you. It doesn't matter if the money never materializes; the thought is enough to give Gary such joy. At night, when Gary falls asleep I swear he's smiling. Before I retire for the night Dr. Carroll pops in. He has a family. What is he doing here? It's not lost on me that he takes the time to come to the hospital this evening. Luckily, I'm still dressed and my contacts are in. Dr. Carroll says there is no need to wake Gary. I sense he just really wants to talk to me. He sits down on the couch. I pull up a chair. Unlike other days, he doesn't seem rushed. I wonder what is on his mind. I sit back on the chair in an open non-threatening position and I let him talk. He starts telling me his life story. He explains to me how he was hospitalized in college and it taught him a big lesson, something that Gary seems to already know: To take advantage of opportunities. He said he didn't do this in high school. As a mother of a boy, especially, I've heard over and over again how it typically takes boys longer to kick into gear. The girls mature faster, and more often will catch on sooner academically. Dr. Carroll lets me know he didn't make Tufts and went to a tier three college instead. I keep listening. I want to see where this conversation is heading and I don't want my thoughts to derail his.

Then he explains about getting into medical school. He offers to talk to Gary about it. He says he will let Gary shadow him at work for a day. I am so grateful for his offer. I don't bring up the fabric. Another time, I figure. As Dr. Carroll gets ready to leave, Gary wakes up. The doctor offers to be Gary's mentor. To Gary, this is on par with potential foundation money.

"Mom, today was a great Thanksgiving," he whispers before falling back to sleep.

Friday morning. Gary wakes up saying he's staying in the

hospital because he needs the morphine. I don't know if I should talk him out of it or what. Steve drives my mom and Matt up for a visit. Fortunately this takes Gary's mind off the drugs and all he talks about is the grant money. He does the math over and over again. If each well pump costs $14,000 and supplies water for 2,600 people, over 16,714 people's lives will change. The thought makes our whole family feel better.

Neither Steve nor I tell Gary that it sounds like a long shot. But, I suspect, Matt's already figured out the low probability of getting so much money so effortlessly. He finds a reason to avoid the obvious questions by claiming he's bored in the room. My mom offers to walk Matt to the game room.

Steve, Gary and I settle in to watch "*Lord of the Rings*" again. Luckily, for me, there is a knock on the door. Dr. Simmon enters and I'm saved from another viewing. I am nervous about Dr. Simmon's visit, though. I fear he won't let Gary return to nutritional therapy now that Gary's had another surgery. The thought of the medications that cause cancer is too much for me to bear. Dr. Simmon takes out photos of Gary's intestine. The doctor studies them but does not show me or my husband. He says nothing. I try to read his facial expressions. Is that a frown? Did he just shake his head? I can tell nothing. What the hell is he here for?

His first words are, "He can stay on nutritional therapy."

Dr. Simmon explains that Gary will be able to eat for three months and then will have to take one month off where he'll just drink nutritional supplements. He'll be able to get an NG tube for home to help him "eat" the liquid food at night. Most people would be terrified of not being able to eat for three months in the year. And then there's that tube again. But, to Gary, it seems better than the alternative.

"So, I can have a pump in my room?"

"Yes, the nurse will teach you how to insert it. You will get a stethoscope to hear if it is inserted properly."

"My own?"

"Yes," Dr. Simmon states.

"When do I start?"

"You'll go home, eat for a month, and then in January you can start," Dr. Simmon explains.

"This is great news," I say as I shake Dr. Simmon's hand. "Doctor, can you talk with my mom as well? She's been anxious about what you'd be saying."

He leaves to talk to my mom. Steve and I stay with Gary. He seems like a new life has been handed to him. My mom comes in and is so excited. "Grandpa is watching out for us," she says. Then she shouts out, "Where are my keys?"

Gary and Matt burst out laughing.

Steve rewards me with a special present − a break. He tells me to drive Matt and Grandma home. He'll stay the night. Just come back on Sunday, he says. I've been here nine days this time. Unlike vacations that are so fun that time flies, this journey was so intense that time stopped. The hospital snatched us away from our world.

Back in Fairfield, I feel the comfort of home. But as I walk in the front door, I sense that the place is the same but I'm not. My view of the world changed. Before, it was comforting for me to place my trust in another person, like a doctor, because it absolved me of responsibility and accountability. But now I know that blind trust can take me down paths I don't want to travel. It is my responsibility to ask "Why" and say "No" if I am not comfortable with the explanation. Standing in my kitchen, I realize I can find out all of the options and gain comfort with the choices I make. This is a lot more work than blind faith. I feel sad for the loss of my innocence. But as the sun pours in the room, I feel a strength return because I am in control. To be my son's best health care advocate, I must look at the entire journey, not just at certain station stops on a hard long track where the choices may seem bleak. Knowledge and acceptance can make moments on the journey more bearable. I must do my best to learn about the entire journey and help prepare my son to navigate it to the best of his ability.

I uncharacteristically decide to go to Shabbat services at our temple. I tell my mom to get her cane and Matt to put on his good shoes and button-down shirt. I usually don't go unless it's a big holiday or a Bar or Bat Mitzvah that I am invited to. My mom never goes. I'm not trained in Judaism. I've never had a Bat Mitzvah. But I know that the rabbi and the congregation pray for the sick. I figure I need all the help I can get.

Turns out, it is Audrey Ross's Bat Mitzvah. I know the parents, but not real well. The parents met at Brandeis, fell in love, had two daughters. He is an attorney and I think she is too. They appear to have a wonderful life. The Rosses adorned the bimah, the podium in the front, with beautiful white and pink flowers. Special velvet yarmulkes were handed out to congregants for the occasion. The 13-year-old wears a new light pink suit. Her father and mother radiate in the glow of their child.

I sit with my mom watching the service. She is crying and I cry too. I'm not sure if I'm happy or sad. The world continues while my son is still in the hospital along with the Indian boy with head trauma, the boy with the fluid on his brain; Cathy's son, the paraplegic with Crohn's; and so many other children in hospitals everywhere. I cry more.

The rabbi stands at the bimah. The Bat Mitzvah is just one part of the service. We remember the sick and people who passed away, a reminder to congregants that the good times are fleeting. I've heard this hundreds of times. Now, I get it.

I wonder how Gary is going to cope with such insight on suffering. I cry some more. I feel weighted down by life's reality, just like when I stood in the African township.

The rabbi approaches my tearful mother and me in our seats, as the Ross family members lead their part of the service.

"Why Gary?" I want to say. "It's not fair," I want to say.

"I have nothing left," is what tumbles out, exposing my soul.

"Yes, you do," he responds.

I hate that answer. Don't tell me I am stronger than I feel. I feel weak. I want to scream, but now is not the time. There is a Bat Mitzvah going on. I take a deep breath. I compose myself and ask the rabbi to add Gary's name to the special prayer for the sick.

As the services proceed, congregants come over and hold my hand or give me a hug. (Services go on for hours; it's not unusual for people to come and go.) I think more people than I realized understand my pain. In the past, many of these people looked troubled to me. Clearly their lives were not perfect. I was too busy to find out more about them, though. I was keeping myself fit, nicely dressed, with wonderful accessories. But, as they hug me tight and look in my eyes, I can tell they understand what my family is going through on a much deeper level. I never realized how clueless I was, maybe even how callous.

The rabbi stands on the bimah to say the prayer for the sick. He says Gary's name first. I feel as if all our souls are praying for him. Now, I understand why we pray together, so we are not alone. I am part of a community.

I drive back to the hospital on Sunday, resolved to help people cope with their own health care crisis and to get my son out of here. When I enter the room, the guys are watching football. If it weren't for the beeping machines, it would be an ordinary Sunday. Gary looks stronger. After the game, Steve kisses us good-bye and goes home. Not long afterwards, I hear a knock on the door. It's not the fast beat triple knock of Dr. Stark and I wonder who is being so formal. I get up and open the door. It is Dr. Carroll, who sits on the couch again. This time, I talk. I tell him how I am concerned about Gary's mental state because he is starting to worry that he is now further behind in school. I let him know how Gary wants to be on the tennis team and that the other kids have been practicing since fall. Dr. Carroll seems to understand that if we could have avoided the second surgery it would have been so much easier on Gary.

Not just the pain, but the mental rollercoaster. I am not sure how much time doctors spend thinking about the person as a whole. But, I am hoping painting this picture of the impact on a patient gives him perspective and he'll think about using the fabric the next time if he can.

Dr. Carroll says he'll help Gary in any way to keep up with school. He stands up to leave and tells me he has another operation to perform. My heart sinks for the family. I hope they do not go through what we've been through.

I ask, "What type of operation?"

"An appendectomy."

"Oh, the kind the fabric may help?" I say.

"Maybe," he says.

"Doctor, if given the chance, do the patient a favor and use the fabric."

He smiles and says, "Point well taken."

What You Can Do Now

---

1. Hug your loved ones.

Life is not a straight line. It is our love that gives each other strength to handle the hurdles.

* * *

Epilogue

Gary got out of the hospital, got tutored again, got caught up in school and even made the junior varsity tennis team his sophomore year. Now he is 19 years old, 5'8" tall and 183 pounds of lean muscle. He is studying nutrition in college and competes in Strongman contests.

He's not currently on any medications and continues to manage his Crohn's with nutritional therapy. Though it's very difficult, twice a year Gary drinks only liquid supplements for three straight weeks. He hopes to learn why this approach is working for him. His mission is to help people live a healthy lifestyle.

Gary eats a mostly gluten-free diet filled with vegetables and lean proteins. He incorporates into his meals ingredients that are inflammation-busters, like cayenne pepper and ginger. Gary minimizes sweets and maximizes exercise. His physique has transformed from skinny kid to muscle-bursting man. He hopes to be a walking example for sick children, showing them they can overcome and achieve in spite of their illness.

Gary has testified on Capitol Hill on behalf of Crohn's patients. He helped create the first national Crohn's awareness week.

He also decided he wanted to help others in health emergencies. After a half dozen ambulance rides he's moved from being a passenger to becoming a nationally certified EMT. He volunteers locally.

Gary's high school club never did receive the $90,000 for water pumps. But the kids hosted enough bake sales, talent shows and

Earth Day events to raise $7,000. Nestlé matched their earnings, bringing the total to $14,000, the amount needed for one pump. The pump was installed in South Africa in June of Gary's junior year of high school.

Gary remembers very few details about his surgery and recovery. For example, when I asked him about the PICC line insertion he said he didn't even realize I was in the room for the procedure. Gary remembers laughing at the Three Stooges on the laptop with his dad before surgery but has no memory of the three days after the surgery.

It's been about four years since his operation. On the positive side, besides him feeling great, the experience matured Gary. He has a perspective about what is truly important, which he attained at a much earlier age than I ever did.

After I was hit by a drunk driver at age 29, and was called in as a possible fatality but survived, I felt I was given a second chance at life. But I often wondered why I was hit. The week before the accident, Steve and I were on a Windjammer vacation. Out in the Atlantic, with the blue sky above as the ship sailed past uninhabited islands, the quiet gave me an epiphany. I wrote in my journal, "Life is a gift, treasure it as you would any other." I closed my journal and felt grateful, as if I was communicating directly to God about how I valued my life. Six days later I found myself lying in the E.R. fighting for my life. It didn't make sense. After a couple of months of recovery, I went right back to my GE job and the pursuit of climbing the corporate ladder. There were days that I'd drive into the office park and sit in my office like it was a prison cell. Even at night when I arrived home, I was still tethered to the office with a modem. I felt empty but filled my house with stuff.

After Gary's recovery, Steve and I decided that I should devote myself to sharing our story to help others. It meant working full time on this memoir, sacrificing my business and the income it produced. I explained to him that I had no idea how the book publishing industry worked and had few contacts who could help me. But, deep inside,

I knew all the experiences that I'd had enabled me to navigate the health care system and to help others. To me, this was one reason why I survived the crash.

Each day I meet more and more people who give me strength to continue to help empower patients to improve their outcomes. I'd love to know how my experience has helped you or your friends and family. Feel free to share your questions, comments and your story with me on my website, **www.RandiRedmondOster.com**. Together we can find a way to affect change for the better in our health care system. Welcome to the team.

Acknowlegments

First I'd like to thank my son, Gary, who, on his hospital bed, watched me type every event into the computer. When I explained to him that his personal story would no longer be private, he said, "Mom, we can help other kids. Go for it!"

I'd also like to thank Matt, who understood I could not be in two places at once and never made me feel bad.

I am indebted to my mom, whose wisdom taught me *to work with what I have and not what I wish for.*

One day I saw a flyer hanging on a bulletin board in the library announcing a writing workshop. I called the teacher, Carol Dannhauser, told her I was an engineer and admitted I couldn't write. She said I was a good storyteller and that she could help me learn the rest. I started taking her classes. Eight years of workshops later, I felt ready to write my memoir and she agreed to be my editor. I am so grateful for her insight, guidance and expertise. But, most important, I am so glad that just as my writing progressed, our relationship did as well. She is a dear friend.

Writing is lonely and hard. Without my friends, like Beatrice Blanco and Jacqueline Danos, I would have given up. They took walks with me, talked with me and kept me focused on my mission to help others. When I complained that I didn't think the book would get out of my basement because I had no idea how to get it published, their belief in me gave me confidence that somehow I'd find a way.

I am grateful to Barbara Lisi, who I already knew as a friend but whose business skills I was unaware of until we worked on my book together. Barbara listened to my story, understood my passion and built my website. She became my branding manager and helped me think big. She helped me because she kept telling me she already loved me. Without her, this book would not have cover art or beauty. Without all of her marketing prowess, you might not have even heard about it. I am grateful to her entire team: Jed Ferdinand, our lawyer; and Fred Iannotti, our publicist.

After I finished writing this memoir, I met respected publishing veteran Gary Krebs at a Fourth of July celebration on the beach. As the sun set, he patiently talked me through the publishing process based on his years of experience, and later introduced me to individuals who could help me continue on my journey. I am grateful to Gary.

As I ventured out to find a way to get the book published I attended a health care conference in Washington D.C. Speaking on the podium was Shannon Brownlee, author of "Overtreated." After our family's experience with Gary, I had read her book, highlighted it and memorized entire portions. Her book confirmed to me the health care system had a process problem. I had to thank her. After her speech, I didn't go around to the stairs on the side of the stage to say hello. I climbed up right in front of her and the 700 members in the audience. I tripped on the microphone. It hit her shoulder. Then I introduced myself as a mom with a way to help others. She looked me right in my eyes and said "I can help you." She has done that ever since.

Thanks to Regina Holliday, an artist who paints patients' stories on jackets so they become a "walking gallery" of stories. One Saturday, Regina took the time to tell me what I needed to do to get my story heard. She offered to paint my story and introduced me to a whole new world of people wanting to improve the health care system. Before Regina, I thought I was a lone wolf. But, I was so wrong. Regina taught me how to get more involved on Twitter and blogs and at conferences. I am grateful that she has become a part of my life.

I am indebted to Anne Llewellyn, an editor at Dorland Health. Anne gave me my first shot as a panelist for a national Webinar, published an excerpt of my story in "Case In Point" and invited me to speak with her at a conference on shared decision-making.

There have been a host of other people in the patient advocacy and business communities that have provided guidance, including Pat Mastors, Dave DeBronkart, Helen Haskell, Jean Rexford and Steve Glick. I am grateful for the compassion and help of the medical community for Gary's care. I found each person was doing their job to the best of their ability and following the current medical protocols.

Finally, eternal thanks to my husband, Steve, whose patience and belief in me gave me the fortitude to not give up writing this book.

Footnotes

1. Slowik, Guy. EhealthMD. Health Information Publications, n.d. Web. May-June 2012. <http://ehealthmd.com/content/how-crohns-disease-treated>.

2. Aspden, Philip, Julie A. Wolcott, J. L. Bootman, and Linda R. Cronenwett, eds. "Preventing Medication Errors." Diss. Institute of Medicine of the National Academies, 2007. Abstract. Preventing Medication Errors: Quality Chasm Series. The National Academies Press, n.d. Web. Aug. 2011. <http://www.nap.edu/openbook. php?record_id=11623>.

3. Demling, Ludwig. "Crohn Disease Caused by Antibiotics? A Medical Hypothesis Based on Epidemiologic Data." Diss. Universität Erlangen-Nürnberg, Schlüsselfeld, 1994. Abstract. National Center for Biotechnology Information. U.S. National Library of Medicine, n.d. Web. Aug. 2011. <http://www.ncbi.nlm.nih.gov/pubmed/8050759>.

4. Card, T. "Antibiotic Use and the Development of Crohn's Disease." GUT - An International Journal of Gastroenterology and Hepatology 53.2 (2004): n. pag. NCBI. PMC - National Library of Medicine, National Institutes of Health. University of Nottingham, Division of Epidemiology and Public Health, Queen's Medical Centre, Nottingham NG7 2UH, UK Web. May-June 2012.< http://gut.bmj.com/content/53/2/246>

5. IBID

6. IBID

7. "Follow-up to the June 4, 2008 Early Communication about the Ongoing Safety Review of Tumor Necrosis Factor (TNF) Blockers (marketed as Remicade, Enbrel, Humira, Cimzia, and Simponi)." Drug Safety and Availability (n.d.): n. pag. Protecting and Promoting Your Health. U.S. Food and Drug Administration, 4 Aug. 2009. Web. Jan. 2011. <http://www.fda.gov/Drugs/DrugSafety/PostmarketDrugSafetyInformationforPatientsandProviders/DrugSafetyInformationforHeathcareProfessionals/ucm174449.htm>.

8. "What Is a PICC Line and Why Do I Need It?" Vascular Access Management. VAM, n.d. Web. Nov. 2009. <http://picclinenursing.com/picc_why.html>.

9. IBID

10. Glower, Michelle Myers. "Six Sigma Convert Offers Views on Healthcare Leadership." ISix Sigma. Michael Cyger, Founder and Publisher, n.d. Web. Apr.-May 2011. <http://www.isixsigma.com/industries/healthcare/six-sigma-convert-offers-views-healthcare-leadership/>.

11. "Six Sigma Quality - Significance of Six Sigma." GE Lighting Solutions. GE Lighting, n.d. Web. 19 Aug. 2012. <http://www.gelightingsolutions.com/education--resources/six-sigma>.

About the Author

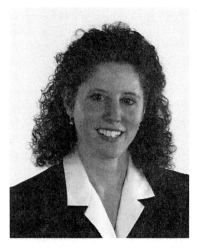 Randi Redmond Oster is an award-winning writer, speaker and expert on health care reform. She worked in the corporate world for about 20 years, specializing in aviation, engineering and finance, prior to starting her own business in the health care industry. Her work – and her life – took a sharp turn during repeated trips to the hospital advocating for her son, who has Crohn's disease.

Randi is a selected member of the Malcolm Baldrige Board of Examiners, focusing on health care. She holds a Bachelor's degree in electrical engineering as well as a Master's of Business Administration.

She lives in Connecticut with her husband, sons and mother.

Reach her at:
www.RandiRedmondOster.com
twitter.com/Protocol123
www.facebook.com/RroAssociates

Sales and Contact Information

Additional copies of **Questioning Protocol**
are available through your favorite
book dealer or from the distributor:

Atlas Books
Phone: (800) 247-6553

Questioning Protocol
ISBN Softbound: 978-0-9899120-0-6 $22.95
(Ask about volume discounts)

If you wish to contact
Randi Redmond Oster:

Randi@RandiRedmondOster.com
Website: www.RandiRedmondOster.com